T0259524

Fatigue

Guest Editors

ADRIAN CRISTIAN, MD
BRIAN D. GREENWALD, MD

PHYSICAL MEDICINE AND REHABILITATION CLINICS OF NORTH AMERICA

www.pmr.theclinics.com

Consulting Editor
GEORGE H. KRAFT, MD, MS

May 2009 • Volume 20 • Number 2

SAUNDERS an imprint of ELSEVIER, Inc.

W.B. SAUNDERS COMPANY
A Division of Elsevier Inc.

1600 John F. Kennedy Boulevard • Suite 1800 • Philadelphia, Pennsylvania 19103

http://www.theclinics.com

PHYSICAL MEDICINE AND REHABILITATION CLINICS OF NORTH AMERICA Volume 20, Number 2
May 2009 ISSN 1047-9651, ISBN-10: 1-4377-0527-8, ISBN-13: 978-1-4377-0527-0

Editor: Debora Dellapena

Reprints. For copies of 100 or more of articles in this publication, please contact the Commercial Reprints Department, Elsevier Inc., 360 Park Avenue South, New York, NY 10010-1710. Tel.: 212-633-3812; Fax: 212-462-1935; E-mail: reprints@elsevier.com.

Physical Medicine and Rehabilitation Clinics of North America (ISSN 1047-9651) is published quarterly by Elsevier Inc., 360 Park Avenue South, New York, NY 10010-1710. Months of publication are February, May, August, and November. Business and Editorial Offices: 1600 John F. Kennedy Blvd., Suite 1800, Philadelphia, PA 19103-2899. Customer Service Office: 11830 Westline Industrial Drive, St. Louis, MO 63146. Periodicals postage paid at New York, NY and additional mailing offices. Subscription price per year is $213.00 (US individuals), $339.00 (US institutions), $107.00 (US students), $259.00 (Canadian individuals), $443.00 (Canadian institutions), $155.00 (Canadian students), $319.00 (foreign individuals), $443.00 (foreign institutions), and $155.00 (foreign students). Foreign air speed delivery is included in all *Clinics* subscription prices. All prices are subject to change without notice. **POSTMASTER:** Send address changes to *Physical Medicine and Rehabilitation Clinics of North America*, Elsevier Periodicals Customer Service, 11830 Westline Industrial Drive, St. Louis, MO 63146. **Customer Service: 1-800-654-2452 (US). From outside of the United States, call 314-453-7041. Fax: 314-453-5170. E-mail: JournalsCustomerService-usa@elsevier.com (for print support); JournalsOnlineSupport-usa@elsevier.com (for online support).**

Physical Medicine and Rehabilitation Clinics of North America is indexed in *Excerpta Medica, MEDLINE/ PubMed (Index Medicus), Cinahl, and Cumulative Index to Nursing and Allied Health Literature.*

Printed and bound by CPI Group (UK) Ltd, Croydon, CR0 4YY

Transferred to Digital Print 2011

Contributors

CONSULTING EDITOR

GEORGE H. KRAFT, MD, MS
Alvord Professor of Multiple Sclerosis Research; Professor, Rehabilitation Medicine; and Adjunct Professor, Neurology, University of Washington School of Medicine, Seattle, Washington

GUEST EDITORS

ADRIAN CRISTIAN, MD
Chief, Rehabilitation Medicine, James J. Peters Veterans Affairs Medical Center; Associate Professor, Department of Rehabilitation Medicine, Mount Sinai School of Medicine, Bronx, New York

BRIAN D. GREENWALD, MD
Assistant Professor of Rehabilitation Medicine, Department of Rehabilitation Medicine, Mount Sinai Medical Center, New York, New York

AUTHORS

MATTHEW N. BARTELS, MD, MPH
John A. Downey Associate Professor of Clinical Rehabilitation Medicine, Department of Rehabilitation Medicine, Columbia College of Physicians and Surgeons, Columbia University, New York, New York

DAVID N. BRESSLER, MD
Assistant Professor, Department of Rehabilitation Medicine, Mount Sinai School of Medicine, New York; Attending Physiatrist, Department of Rehabilitation Medicine, Elmhurst Hospital Center, Elmhurst, New York

EMLYN J. CAPILI, BA
Graduate School of Biomedical Science, University of Medicine and Dentistry of New Jersey – New Jersey Medical School, Newark, New Jersey

JAISHREE CAPOOR, MD, FAAP
The Mount Sinai School of Medicine, Elmhurst Hospital, Blythedale Children's Hospital, Elmhurst, New York

ANDREA L. CHEVILLE, MD, MSCE
Associate Professor of Physical Medicine and Rehabilitation, Mayo Clinic, Rochester, Minnesota

ADRIAN CRISTIAN, MD
Chief, Rehabilitation Medicine, James J. Peters Veterans Affairs Medical Center; Associate Professor, Department of Rehabilitation Medicine, Mount Sinai School of Medicine, Bronx, New York

JOHN DeLUCA, PhD, ABPP
Vice President for Research, Kessler Foundation Research Center, West Orange; Professor of Physical Medicine and Rehabilitation, Department of Physical and Rehabilitation; and Professor of Neurology and Neuroscience, University of Medicine and Dentistry of New Jersey – New Jersey Medical School, Newark, New Jersey

HELEN M. GENOVA, PhD
Research Associate, Kessler Foundation Research Center, West Orange, New Jersey

BRIAN D. GREENWALD, MD
Assistant Professor of Rehabilitation Medicine, Department of Rehabilitation Medicine, Mount Sinai Medical Center, New York, New York

RAJ K. KALAPATAPU, MD
Fellow, Geriatric Psychiatry, Mount Sinai School of Medicine, New York, New York

MICHELLE KARCZEWSKI, MD
Department of Rehabilitation Medicine, New York-Presbyterian Hospital, Weill Cornell Medical Center, New York, New York

JAIME LEVINE, DO
Chief Resident, Department of Physical Medicine and Rehabilitation, St. Vincent's Medical Center, New York, New York

MARYKATHARINE NUTINI, DO
The Mount Sinai Hospital, Department of Rehabilitation Medicine, New York, New York

JOHN C. PAN, MD
Resident Physician, Department of Rehabilitation Medicine, Mount Sinai School of Medicine, Mount Sinai Medical Center, New York, New York

ANJALI SHAH, MD
Director of Multiple Sclerosis Neurorehabilitation, Assistant Professor, Department of Physical Medicine and Rehabilitation, University of Texas Southwestern Medical Center, Dallas, Texas

GLENN R. WYLIE, DPhil
Research Scientist, Kessler Foundation Research Center, West Orange; Associate Professor of Physical Medicine and Rehabilitation, University of Medicine and Dentistry of New Jersey – New Jersey Medical School, Newark, New Jersey

Contents

Andrea L. Cheville

> Up to 50% of Americans will develop cancer, and >90% of patients will experience cancer-related fatigue (CRF) at some point in their disease course. Patients describe CRF as devastating to many life domains, degrading their vocational, familial, and societal roles. This article describes current best efforts to define CRF and to characterize its epidemiology using these definitions. In addition, the article will outlines assessment tools, proposed mechanisms, associated symptoms, and treatment strategies. Readers are offered highly more comprehensive references relating to specific aspects of CRF throughout.

THE CLINICS ARE NOW AVAILABLE ONLINE!

Access your subscription at:
www.theclinics.com

Foreword

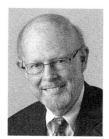

George H. Kraft, MD, MS
Consulting Editor

There was a time when fatigue was not considered to be an intrinsic part of any disease. It was something almost everyone complained of at one time or another, so how could it be part of a disease? Yes, fatigue was seen in medical conditions, but it was considered to be a nonspecific result of the deterioration associated with many chronic conditions. Fatigue was thought to be an inevitable consequence of lack of sleep, too much work, excessive physical activity, inadequate diet, boredom, stress, depression, the catabolism of a chronic medical condition, or the effect of medications. In medicine and physiology it was used primarily to describe the exhaustion of muscle with tetanic stimulation.[1] But fatigue was not a fundamental component of any disease.

That changed in early 1984 with our publication of "Symptomatic fatigue in multiple sclerosis."[2] In this article we reported that disabling fatigue was a common symptom of multiple sclerosis (MS). We found it to be the *most* prevalent MS symptom, and seen in patients across the entire disability spectrum. It was a fundamental part of the disease. To my knowledge, this was the first report of fatigue as an inherent part of any disease.

So it was with great enthusiasm that I welcomed the offer by Dr. Adrian Cristian to guest-edit, with his colleague Dr. Brian Greenwald, an issue of the *Physical Medicine and Rehabilitation Clinics of North America* on fatigue. Dr. Cristian has worked with us previously in 2005 as guest editor of an issue on aging with a disability.[3] This issue of the *Clinics* on fatigue is being published 25 years after the first description of fatigue as intrinsic to a disease process. Over that period of time, the medical awareness of fatigue has grown and much has been learned about it being intrinsic to other diseases as well. In the 1990s my rheumatologist friends talked about fatigue being intrinsic to rheumatoid arthritis too. So it is good to see an article in this issue on fatigue in rheumatologic diseases by Drs. Pan and Bressler. I have mentioned earlier about fatigue in MS, and it is especially gratifying to see an article reviewing this topic by one of my previous MS fellows, Dr. Shah.

Fatigue in other medical conditions is also discussed: Parkinson's disease, stroke, and traumatic brain injury by Drs. Levine and Greenwald, cardiopulmonary disease

Phys Med Rehabil Clin N Am 20 (2009) ix–x
doi:10.1016/j.pmr.2009.03.001

by Dr. Bartels, and cancer by Dr. Cheville. Fatigue in adults is discussed by Drs. Kalapatapu and Cristian and fatigue in children with neurologic impairments by Drs. Nutini, Karczewski, and Capoor. Finally, there is an article on functional neuroimaging of fatigue by Drs. DeLuca, Genova, Capili, and Wylie.

There are many theories about the causes of fatigue seen in various medical conditions. I suspect that there are many factors explaining fatigue, and that they may be quite different in different conditions. This issue of the *Clinics* will serve as a good up-to-date reference on this topic.

George H. Kraft, MD, MS
Department of Rehabilitation Medicine
University of Washington
Box 356490, 1959 NE Pacific Street
Seattle, WA 98195-6490, USA

E-mail address:
ghkraft@u.washington.edu (G.H. Kraft)

REFERENCES

1. Young JL, Mayer RF. Physiological alterations of motor units in hemiplegia. J Neurol Sci 1982;54(3):401–12.
2. Freal JE, Kraft GH, Coryell JK. Symptomatic fatigue in multiple sclerosis. Arch Phys Med Rehabil 1984;65:135–8.
3. Cristian A, editor. Aging with a disability. Phys Med Rehabil Clin N Am 2005;16(4).

Preface

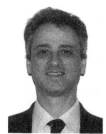 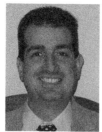

Adrian Cristian, MD   Brian D. Greenwald, MD
Guest Editors

Medical literature generally defines fatigue as an overwhelming sense of tiredness, lack of energy, and feeling of exhaustion. Although there is no universally accepted definition for fatigue, there is a general distinction between central and peripheral fatigue. Central fatigue has the key component of inability to maintain focused attention, whereas peripheral fatigue is expressed as reduced exercise tolerance.

Although fatigue is seen in 10% to 20% of the general population, it is reported at much higher rates across a large spectrum of diseases and disorders commonly seen by physical medicine and rehabilitation specialists. Fatigue is a primary or significant cause of disability in many disease processes. The spectrum of these diseases includes central nervous system disorders, cardiopulmonary disorders, and rheumatologic disorders. Fatigue is often reported as the primary symptom at the time of diagnosis and as the most troubling symptom in patients with multiple sclerosis and chronic fatigue syndrome. More than 90% of patients with cancer will experience fatigue during the course of their disease.[1]

In addition to the nebulous qualities of its definition and measurement, the pathophysiology of fatigue remains elusive, and evaluation often revolves around ruling out and treating co-morbid conditions that cause or worsen this pervasive disorder. Advances in neuroradiology are also expanding our understanding of the structures in the brain that underlie fatigue. Treatment generally involves pharmacologic and rehabilitation interventions tailored to the patient's needs and goals.

This issue of the *Physical Medicine and Rehabilitation Clinics of North America* is devoted to this important topic. Subjects covered include the assessment, presentation, and treatment of fatigue in adults with various disorders, such as multiple sclerosis, spinal cord injury, traumatic brain injury, rheumatologic disorders, and

Phys Med Rehabil Clin N Am 20 (2009) xi–xii
doi:10.1016/j.pmr.2009.02.001
1047-9651/09/$ – see front matter © 2009 Elsevier Inc. All rights reserved.

pmr.theclinics.com

cardiopulmonary disorders. Additional topics covered include neuroimaging of fatigue and fatigue in children.

Adrian Cristian, MD
Department of Rehabilitation Medicine
3d-22, James J. Peters Veterans Affairs Medical Center
130 W. Kingsbridge Road
Bronx, NY 10468, USA
Department of Rehabilitation Medicine
Mount Sinai School of Medicine, USA

Brian D. Greenwald, MD
Department of Rehabilitation Medicine
Mount Sinai Medical Center
5 East 98th Street
Box 1240B
New York, NY 10029, USA

E-mail addresses:
acristianmd@msn.com (A. Cristian)
brian.greenwald@mountsinai.org (B.D. Greenwald)

REFERENCE

1. Curt GA, Breitbart W, Cella D, et al. Impact of cancer-related fatigue on the lives of patients: new findings from the Fatigue Coalition. Oncologist 2000;5(5):353–60.

Assessment of Fatigue in Adults with Disabilities

Raj K. Kalapatapu, MD[a],*, Adrian Cristian, MD[b]

KEYWORDS

• Fatigue • Etiology • Adult • Rating scale • Assessment

Clinical fatigue has been described to include 3 major features: (1) generalized weakness, causing an inability to begin certain activities, (2) easy fatigability and decreased ability to maintain performance, and (3) mental fatigue, resulting in memory loss, impaired concentration, and emotional lability.[1] Based on the duration of symptoms, fatigue can be categorized into 3 categories: (1) recent fatigue—symptoms lasting less than 1 month, (2) prolonged fatigue—symptoms lasting more than 1 month, and (3) chronic fatigue—symptoms lasting greater than 6 months but not automatically implying chronic fatigue syndrome.[2]

Patients with a chief complaint of fatigue are frequently encountered by physicians across the world. In a postal survey of 6 general practices in southern England, 18.3% of respondents reported substantial fatigue lasting 6 months or longer.[3] In a rural family medicine clinic in Israel, almost 32% of adult patients reported symptoms of fatigue or its equivalent terms at least once during a 10-year period.[4] In a representative study of adults in the United States, 14.3% of male respondents and 20.4% of female respondents reported suffering from fatigue.[5] Studies from Canada[6] and France[7] have reported similar findings.

Fatigue can produce serious public health consequences. In a study of the elderly from Norway, physical fatigue represented a possible risk factor for falls.[8] In a US study estimating fatigue prevalence and associated health-related lost productive time (LPT), workers with fatigue annually cost employers $136.4 billion in health-related LPT, representing an excess of $101.0 billion compared with workers without

Dr. Kalapatapu has no competing financial interests.
Dr. Cristian has no competing financial interests.
[a] Geriatric Psychiatry, Mount Sinai School of Medicine, One Gustave L. Levy Place, Box 1230, New York, NY 10029, USA
[b] Department of Rehabilitation Medicine, Mount Sinai School of Medicine, 526/117 Room 3d-16, James J. Peters Veterans Affairs Medical Center, 130 W. Kingsbridge Road, Bronx, NY 10468, USA
* Corresponding author.
E-mail address: rajkumar.kalapatapu@mssm.edu (R.K. Kalapatapu).

Phys Med Rehabil Clin N Am 20 (2009) 313–324
doi:10.1016/j.pmr.2008.12.001
1047-9651/08/$ – see front matter © 2009 Elsevier Inc. All rights reserved.

fatigue.[9] Fatigue represents anywhere from 7 to 10 million office visits to physicians per year.[10,11]

Fatigue has a variety of etiologies (**Fig. 1**). In a prospective cohort study of members of a health maintenance organization, medical or psychiatric disorders accounted for 66% of patients who reported chronic fatigue.[12] In a series of 217 patients presenting with a complaint of fatigue, 35% had endocrine, cardiovascular, respiratory, or hematologic causes, and 65% had psychiatric causes.[13] In a retrospective chart review of 176 patients with a diagnosis of fatigue during a 12-month period, 39% were caused by physical causes, 41% were caused by psychological causes, and 12% were caused by mixed causes.[14]

Fatigue is commonly associated with both physical illness and psychiatric disorders.[15,16] Careful clinical assessment is required to determine the presence of any underlying disorder(s) that may lead to fatigue, although the cause may not always be identified. In a study of final diagnoses in patients presenting to Dutch family physicians, a specific diagnosis was not identified in 37.5% of patients who presented with general weakness or tiredness.[17]

The goal of this review article is to discuss how the physical medicine and rehabilitation (PM&R) physician might assess fatigue in an adult patient with disabilities.

ASSESSMENT OF FATIGUE

The clinical assessment of fatigue begins before the patient even enters the physician's office. Simply observing and talking to the patient while going from the waiting room to the office may reveal a wealth of information. Does she independently get up from a chair? Is he using crutches? Is her speech dysarthric? Is his affect flat? Does she become short of breath? Is he lethargic? Is she using a wheelchair? Does he cough? Does she have a cast? Does he fall? Early attention to such details starts the process of formulating a differential diagnosis, long before any complex physical examination, expensive laboratory studies, or lengthy rating scales.

Obtaining a thorough history of the fatigue from the patient is important, as the medical history sets the tone for the remainder of the assessment. Important information includes date of onset, duration, frequency, aggravating factors, relieving factors, and associated symptoms. It is also important to ask about the impact of fatigue on activities of daily living such as ambulation, transfers from different surfaces, dressing, bathing, meal preparation, work, and hobbies.

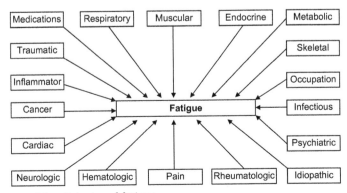

Fig. 1. Some possible etiologies of fatigue.

As often as possible, the patient's own words should be documented in the medical record using quotes. Collateral information from a family member or other caregiver is especially critical when a patient is cognitively impaired. Documenting items such as a review of systems, current prescribed medications (**Box 1**), over-the-counter medications, medical illnesses, surgical history, trauma history, psychiatric history, substance use history, family history, occupational history, and living environment can help paint a well-rounded clinical picture of the patient. A review of any prior medical records can provide additional collateral information.

Many unidimensional and multidimensional rating scales are available for the assessment of fatigue,[18] which may be valuable in further characterization of the fatigue (**Box 2**). A particular rating scale must be carefully chosen based on multiple factors, such as what aspects of fatigue are to be assessed and the specific patient population in which the scale has been validated.[18]

The physical examination begins with measuring vital signs. Is she tachypneic? Does he have a fever? Is she hypotensive? What is his pain rating? Before using any elaborate instruments, gross observations with the naked eye should be made. How is her gait? Are his lips blue? Does she have all limbs? Are his eyes yellow? In an orderly manner, each organ system should be evaluated, noting pertinent positive and negative findings. A thorough neurologic and orthopedic examination is very important as is a functional assessment of the patient's ability to rise from the seated position and ambulate. Special note should be made of the amount of assistance that the patient requires for these activities.

Based on the information obtained thus far, a reasonable differential diagnosis for fatigue can be formulated at this juncture. Appropriate laboratory studies should be ordered only after obtaining a detailed history and physical examination. There is no "routine" laboratory workup for fatigue, as each patient's history, physical examination, and differential diagnosis are unique. Laboratory studies ought to be viewed as complementary to—not substituting for—a comprehensive history and physical examination.

ETIOLOGIES OF FATIGUE

Although each category is discussed separately, the PM&R physician must remember that in a given patient, fatigue may be explained by more than 1 etiology at a certain

---

Box 1
Medications that may cause fatigue[2,19-21]

Beta blockers

Angiotensin-converting enzyme inhibitors

Sedative-hypnotics

Antipsychotics

Antidepressants

Anticonvulsants

Antispasticity drugs

Chemotherapeutic drugs

Interferon

Anesthetics

Analgesics

Box 2
Examples of scales measuring fatigue[18,23,30,63,64]

Fatigue Severity Scale

Visual Analog Scale for Fatigue

Barrow Neurologic Institute Fatigue Scale

Cause of Fatigue Questionnaire

Fatigue Impact Scale

Barroso Fatigue Scale

Fatigue Descriptive Scale

Myasthenia Gravis Fatigue Scale

Task-Induced Fatigue Scale

Chronic Respiratory Disease Questionnaire

Fatigue Assessment Instrument

Brief Mental Fatigue Questionnaire

Rhoten Fatigue Scale

Fatigue Symptom Inventory

FibroFatigue Scale

Dutch Exertion Fatigue Scale

Revised-Piper Fatigue Scale

Schwartz Cancer Fatigue Scale

point in time. Furthermore, just because 1 etiology is found, it does not mean that the search for other contributing etiologies should be halted. Each category includes a discussion of clinical disorders that may present with fatigue and common methods used to diagnose fatigue in the presence of these disorders.

Iatrogenic

A thorough review of all prescribed medications by all physicians from whom the patient is seeking care is warranted at every visit. Many medications, especially when first administered, may cause fatigue (**Table 1**).[2,19–21] These include, but are not limited to, beta blockers, angiotensin-converting enzyme inhibitors, sedative-hypnotics, antipsychotics, antidepressants, anticonvulsants, antispasticity drugs, chemotherapeutic drugs, interferon, anesthetics, or analgesics. The continued medical indication for each medication should be analyzed at every appointment. If medically feasible, an effort should be made to discontinue or minimize the number of such medications contributing to fatigue.

Traumatic

Fatigue is common in patients with spinal cord injury and traumatic brain injury (TBI). Prevalence of fatigue ranges from 50% to 80% in patients with TBI living in the community. Etiologies of trauma include, but are not limited to, motor vehicle accidents, violence, or falls. Imaging studies, such as computed tomography (CT), magnetic resonance imaging (MRI), or x-ray, may be helpful in the diagnosis of traumatic disorders. One scale used to assess fatigue in the presence of TBI is the Barroso

Table 1 Internet resources on fatigue	
National Library of Medicine/National Institutes of Health	http://www.nlm.nih.gov/MEDLINEPLUS/ency/article/003088.htm
National Cancer Institute	http://www.cancer.gov/cancertopics/pdq/supportivecare/fatigue/Patient
American Cancer Society	http://www.cancer.org/docroot/MIT/MIT_2_2x_Fatigue.asp
Muscular Dystrophy Association	http://www.mda.org/publications/Quest/q121fatigue.html
Mayo Clinic	http://www.mayoclinic.com/health/fatigue/HQ00673
University of Maryland	http://www.umm.edu/ency/article/003088.htm
University of Texas	http://www.mdanderson.org/topics/fatigue/
AIDS InfoNet—University of New Mexico	http://www.aidsinfonet.org/fact_sheets/view/551
eMedicine Health	http://www.emedicinehealth.com/fatigue/article_em.htm

Fatigue Scale, which was created from 5 other fatigue scales: Multidimensional Assessment for Fatigue, Fatigue Severity Scale, Fatigue Assessment Instrument, Fatigue Impact Scale, and General Fatigue Scale.[22–24] The Fatigue Severity Scale has been used to assess fatigue in patients with spinal cord injury.[25]

Inflammatory

Inflammatory etiologies of fatigue include, but are not limited to, systemic lupus erythematosus (SLE), rheumatoid arthritis,[26] and ankylosing spondylitis. Laboratory studies, such as erythrocyte sedimentation rate, antinuclear antibody, or rheumatoid factor, may be helpful in the diagnosis of inflammatory disorders. A working group and expert panel on SLE has recommended the 9-item Fatigue Severity Scale for the assessment of fatigue in patients with SLE.[27] The Multidimensional Assessment for Fatigue Scale has been used to assess fatigue in patients with ankylosing spondylitis.[28]

Neurologic

Neurologic etiologies of fatigue include, but are not limited to, multiple sclerosis (MS), stroke, motor neuron disease,[29] or myasthenia gravis. Cranial nerve, sensory, reflex, strength, or focal abnormalities may be uncovered with a thorough neurologic examination. Laboratory studies, such as head CT, head MRI, electromyography, cerebrospinal spinal fluid analysis, or the Tensilon test, may be helpful in the diagnosis of neurologic disorders. Scales such as the Fatigue Severity Scale, the Fatigue Impact Scale, the Fatigue Descriptive Scale, and the Task Induced Fatigue Scale have been used in the assessment of MS-related fatigue.[30,31] The Fatigue Impact Scale and the Checklist Individual Strength (fatigue subscale) have been used in the assessment of post-stroke fatigue.[32] The Myasthenia Gravis Fatigue Scale has been used in the assessment of myasthenia gravis-related fatigue.[33]

Psychiatric

Depressive disorders such as major depressive disorder can lead to fatigue. A major depressive episode is defined by the Diagnostic and Statistical Manual of Mental Disorders, 4th Edition, Text Revision (DSM-IV-TR),[34] as a 2-week period of 5 or more of the following symptoms: depressed mood, diminished interest in activities, weight loss, sleep changes, fatigue, feelings of worthlessness, psychomotor agitation/retardation, poor concentration, and recurrent thoughts of death. The symptoms must cause significant impairment in important areas of functioning and not be due to the direct physiologic effects or a substance or a general medical condition. On mental status examination, assessment of appearance, behavior, mood, affect, and safety can be helpful in making a diagnosis of major depressive disorder. The Hamilton Depression Rating Scale, the Beck Depression Inventory-II, and the Montgomery-Asberg Depression Rating Scale can be used to assess fatigue in patients with major depressive disorder.[35]

Anxiety disorders, such as generalized anxiety disorder (GAD), can lead to fatigue. DSM-IV-TR criteria for GAD include excessive anxiety and worry about a number of events or activities, difficulty controlling the worry, restlessness, being easily fatigued, difficulty concentrating, irritability, muscle tension, and sleep disturbance.[34] The symptoms must cause significant impairment in important areas of functioning and not be due to the direct physiologic effects or a substance or a general medical condition. On mental status examination, assessment of appearance, psychomotor abnormalities, mood, and affect can be helpful in making a diagnosis of GAD. The Worry and Anxiety Questionnaire is based on DSM criteria for GAD and includes questions about the associated somatic symptoms of GAD.[36]

When fatigue is present, substance use disorders should be considered. Patients with chronic fatigue and a lifetime history of a substance use disorder have been reported to have more lifetime symptoms of depression and are more likely to have a history of suicidal ideations or attempts.[37] DSM-IV-TR criteria for substance abuse include recurrent substance use resulting in a failure to fulfill major role obligations, use in physically hazardous situations, substance-related legal problems, or use despite persistent or recurrent social or interpersonal problems caused or exacerbated by the effects of the substance.[34] DSM-IV-TR criteria for substance dependence include tolerance, withdrawal, using in larger amounts or longer than intended, unsuccessful efforts to cut down use, great deal of time spent in activities needed to obtain the substance, important activities given up or reduced due to substance use, or use despite knowledge of having a physical or psychological problem likely to have been caused or exacerbated by the substance.[34] Laboratory studies, such as a urine toxicology screen, can be helpful in detecting use of cocaine, amphetamines, cannabis, opiates, and benzodiazepines. Alcohol use disorders can be screened with questionnaires such as the CAGE questionnaire, the Michigan Alcohol Screening Test, and the Alcohol Use Disorders Identification Test. Laboratory studies, such as liver function tests (aspartate transaminase, alanine transaminase), mean corpuscular volume, gamma-glutamyl transpeptidase, and carbohydrate-deficient transferrin, can also be helpful in detecting alcohol use disorders.

Neuromuscular

Neuromuscular disorders such as facioscapulohumeral dystrophy, myotonic dystrophy, or hereditary motor and sensory neuropathy can lead to fatigue. Patients may complain of weakness of muscles, stiffness, cognitive problems, cold feet, muscle pain, dysphagia, respiratory insufficiency, or loss of balance. Physical examination may reveal muscle wasting, ptosis, weakness in various muscles of the body, foot deformities, foot drop, sensory abnormalities, or reflex abnormalities. Laboratory studies, such as creatine kinase levels, genetic testing, muscle biopsy, nerve biopsy, cerebrospinal fluid analysis, or a nerve conduction study, may be helpful in the diagnosis of neuromuscular disorders. The Checklist Individual Strength scale has been used in the assessment of fatigue in patients with neuromuscular disorders.[38]

Pain

Pain disorders such as fibromyalgia can lead to fatigue. Symptoms may include widespread pain, muscle aches, muscle spasms, sleep disturbances, allodynia, or headaches. Findings on physical examination include tenderness in 11 of 18 point sites on digital palpation.[39] The Fibromyalgia Impact Questionnaire,[40,41] the Multidimensional Fatigue Inventory,[42] and the FibroFatigue Scale[43] have been used to assess fatigue in patients with fibromyalgia.

Respiratory

Fatigue may be caused by respiratory disorders such as chronic obstructive pulmonary disease, obstructive sleep apnea, or sarcoidosis. A detailed physical examination may yield abnormal signs such as wheezing, red bumps on the skin, or swollen lymph nodes. Laboratory studies, such as a chest x-ray, chest CT, pulmonary function tests, bronchoscopy, or polysomnography, may be helpful in the diagnosis of respiratory disorders. The Fatigue Assessment Scale has been used in the assessment of sarcoidosis-related fatigue.[44] The Multidimensional Fatigue Inventory has been used to assess fatigue in patients with chronic obstructive pulmonary disease,[45] and the Chronic Respiratory Disease questionnaire contains items assessing fatigue.[46] The Fatigue Severity Scale has been used in the assessment of fatigue related to sleep disorders.[47]

Cancer

Fatigue in patients with cancer may be related to multiple factors, including the underlying neoplasm itself, antineoplastic treatments, coexisting systemic diseases, electrolyte abnormalities, endocrine abnormalities, chronic pain, deconditioning, sleep disorders, depression, or anxiety.[48–50] Findings on history and physical examination such as cachexia, night sweats, unusual lumps, or hemoptysis may raise suspicion for an underlying neoplastic process. Laboratory studies, such as a complete blood cell count, CT, MRI, or a biopsy, may expose a cancer. Scales that have been used to assess cancer-related fatigue include the Fatigue Assessment Questionnaire, Multidimensional Fatigue Inventory, Fatigue Symptom Inventory, Functional Assessment of Cancer Therapy (Fatigue subscale), Linear Analog Fatigue Scale, Revised-Piper Fatigue Scale, Rhoten Fatigue Scale, Pearson-Byars Fatigue Feeling Checklist, Visual Analog Fatigue Scale, Cancer Fatigue Scale, and Revised Schwartz Cancer Fatigue Scale.[51–53]

Infectious

Infectious etiologies of fatigue include, but are not limited to, influenza, infectious mononucleosis, pneumonia, Lyme disease, Human immunodeficiency virus, or parasitic diseases. Manifestations of an infectious process may consist of fever, chills, cough, headache, malaise, or headache. A physical examination may discover rales, lymphadenopathy, rash, or sore throat. Laboratory studies, such as a complete blood cell count, monospot test, chest x-ray, urinalysis, cerebrospinal fluid analysis, viral titer, stool culture, or blood culture, may be helpful in diagnosing an infectious disorder. The Daily Fatigue Impact Scale has been used to assess fatigue in patients with an influenza-like illness.[54] The Fatigue Assessment Instrument has been used to assess fatigue in patients with Lyme disease and post-Lyme chronic fatigue.[55]

Hepatic

Hepatic etiologies of fatigue include, but are not limited to, primary biliary cirrhosis, primary sclerosing cholangitis, or hepatitis C. Treatments for hepatitis such as interferon may also lead to fatigue. Symptoms of hepatic disease include loss of appetite, dark urine, or abdominal discomfort. Jaundice, hepatomegaly, or splenomegaly may be found on physical examination. Laboratory studies, such as liver function tests, viral antigens/antibodies, antimitochondrial antibodies, abdominal ultrasound, or abdominal CT, may be helpful in the diagnosis of hepatic disorders. The Fatigue Impact Scale has been used to assess fatigue in patients with primary biliary cirrhosis[56] and primary sclerosing cholangitis.[57] The Multidimensional Assessment of Fatigue Scale has been used to assess fatigue in patients with hepatitis C.[58]

Renal

Factors that may lead to fatigue in patients with renal disorders such as end-stage renal disease include prescribed medications, abnormal urea and hemoglobin values, sleep disorders, and psychological factors such as depression.[59,60] The Fatigue Severity Scale,[59] the Short-Form Health Survey vitality subscale, and the Revised-Piper Fatigue Scale have been used to assess fatigue in patients with end-stage renal disease.[60]

Endocrine

Endocrine causes of fatigue may include hypothyroidism, diabetes mellitus, pituitary insufficiency, or adrenal insufficiency. Symptoms of endocrine disorders may include weight loss, loss of appetite, depression, muscle cramps, cold intolerance, polyuria, polydipsia, or polyphagia. Laboratory studies, such as electrolytes, thyroid-stimulating hormone, fasting blood glucose, glycosylated hemoglobin, serum cortisol, or serum aldosterone, may be helpful in the diagnosis of endocrine disorders. The Fatigue Questionnaire has been used to assess fatigue in patients with Addison's disease.[61]

Cardiovascular

Cardiovascular etiologies of fatigue include, but are not limited to, congestive heart failure and pulmonary hypertension. Symptoms may include dyspnea on exertion, dyspnea at rest, orthopnea, paroxysmal nocturnal dyspnea, or exercise intolerance. Edema, hepatomegaly, rales, heart murmurs, or cyanosis may be found on physical examination. Laboratory studies, such as echocardiography, chest x-ray, or electrocardiography, may be helpful in the diagnosis of cardiovascular disorders. The Fatigue Assessment Scale and the Dutch Exertion Fatigue Scale have been used to assess fatigue in patients with heart failure.[62]

Others

Fatigue may result from a wide variety of other etiologies, such as hematologic disorders (eg, severe anemia), metabolic disorders (eg, hypercalcemia), excessive physical activity, insomnia, jet lag, and somatization disorder. A careful history, a thorough physical examination, and pertinent laboratory studies will help clarify which etiology or etiologies may be contributing to a patient's fatigue.

INFORMATION ON FATIGUE FOR PATIENTS

Given the prevalence of fatigue and the plethora of etiologies, educating patients about fatigue is important. Informing patients that they are not alone can be the first step to opening a discussion about fatigue and the impact on one's life. Creating a comfortable and nonjudgmental atmosphere during an appointment can help facilitate the patient in expressing his/her experience with fatigue. Internet resources that contain patient-friendly printable information about fatigue are listed in **Table 1**. Patients can also be informed about the existence of a medical journal dedicated to fatigue called the International Journal of Fatigue, highlighting the medical profession's recognition of this important symptom.

SUMMARY

Fatigue is prevalent and can produce major public health consequences. Assessment of fatigue by the PM&R physician begins with a careful history and physical examination, complemented by pertinent rating scales and laboratory studies. In adults with disabilities, a wide variety of etiologies may lead to fatigue. Educating and providing resources about fatigue to patients can help open the discussion about this highly debilitating symptom.

REFERENCES

1. Markowitz AJ, Rabow MW. Palliative management of fatigue at the close of life: "it feels like my body is just worn out". JAMA 2007;298(2):217.
2. Fosnocht KM, Ende J. UpToDate: approach to the adult patient with fatigue; 2008. Accessed September 10, 2008.
3. Pawlikowska T, Chalder T, Hirsch SR, et al. Population based study of fatigue and psychological distress. BMJ 1994;308(6931):763–6.
4. Shahar E, Lederer J. Asthenic symptoms in a rural family practice. Epidemiologic characteristics and a proposed classification. J Fam Pract 1990;31(3):257–61 [discussion: 261–2].
5. Chen MK. The epidemiology of self-perceived fatigue among adults. Prev Med 1986;15(1):74–81.
6. Cathebras PJ, Robbins JM, Kirmayer LJ, et al. Fatigue in primary care: prevalence, psychiatric comorbidity, illness behavior, and outcome. J Gen Intern Med 1992;7(3):276–86.
7. Fuhrer R, Wessely S. The epidemiology of fatigue and depression: a French primary-care study. Psychol Med 1995;25(5):895–905.
8. Helbostad JL, Leirfall S, Moe-Nilssen R, et al. Physical fatigue affects gait characteristics in older persons. J Gerontol A Biol Sci Med Sci 2007;62(9):1010–5.
9. Ricci JA, Chee E, Lorandeau AL, et al. Fatigue in the U.S. workforce: prevalence and implications for lost productive work time. J Occup Environ Med 2007;49(1): 1–10.
10. Cypress BK. Office visits to internists: the National Ambulatory Medical Care Survey, United States, 1975. Vital Health Stat 13 1978;(36):1–70.
11. Schappert SM. National Ambulatory Medical Care Survey: 1989 summary. Vital Health Stat 13 1992;(110):1–80.
12. Buchwald D, Umali P, Umali J, et al. Chronic fatigue and the chronic fatigue syndrome: prevalence in a Pacific Northwest health care system. Ann Intern Med 1995;123(2):81–8.

13. Gilbert JR. Highlights from a recent seminar on fatigue. Can Med Assoc J 1971; 105(3):309–10.

14. Morrison JD. Fatigue as a presenting complaint in family practice. J Fam Pract 1980;10(5):795–801.

15. Watanabe N, Stewart R, Jenkins R, et al. The epidemiology of chronic fatigue, physical illness, and symptoms of common mental disorders: a cross-sectional survey from the second British National Survey of Psychiatric Morbidity. J Psychosom Res 2008;64(4):357–62.

16. Wijeratne C, Hickie I, Brodaty H. The characteristics of fatigue in an older primary care sample. J Psychosom Res 2007;62(2):153–8.

17. Okkes IM, Oskam SK, Lamberts H. The probability of specific diagnoses for patients presenting with common symptoms to Dutch family physicians. J Fam Pract 2002;51(1):31–6.

18. Dittner AJ, Wessely SC, Brown RG. The assessment of fatigue: a practical guide for clinicians and researchers. J Psychosom Res 2004;56(2):157–70.

19. Lim W, Thomas KS, Dimsdale JE. Chapter 27: pain management, psychological factors and cancer pain—fatigue and cancer pain. In: Lichtman MA, Beutler E, Kipps TJ, et al, editors. Williams hematology. New York: The McGraw-Hill Companies; 2006.

20. O'Rourke RA, Shaver JA, Silverman ME. Chapter 12: the history, physical examination, and cardiac auscultation. In: Walsh RA, Simon DI, Hoit BD, et al, editors. Hurst's the heart. New York: The McGraw-Hill Companies; 2008.

21. Ropper AH, Brown RH. Chapter 24: fatigue, asthenia, anxiety, and depressive reactions - fatigue and asthenia. In: Ropper AH, Brown RH, editors. Adams and Victor's Principles of Neurology. 8th edition. New York: The McGraw-Hill Companies; 2005.

22. Bushnik T, Englander J, Katznelson L. Fatigue after TBI: association with neuroendocrine abnormalities. Brain Inj 2007;21(6):559–66.

23. Bushnik T, Englander J, Wright J. Patterns of fatigue and its correlates over the first 2 years after traumatic brain injury. J Head Trauma Rehabil 2008;23(1):25–32.

24. Bushnik T, Englander J, Wright J. The experience of fatigue in the first 2 years after moderate-to-severe traumatic brain injury: a preliminary report. J Head Trauma Rehabil 2008;23(1):17–24.

25. Fawkes-Kirby TM, Wheeler MA, Anton HA, et al. Clinical correlates of fatigue in spinal cord injury. Spinal Cord 2008;46(1):21–5.

26. Hewlett S, Cockshott Z, Byron M, et al. Patients' perceptions of fatigue in rheumatoid arthritis: overwhelming, uncontrollable, ignored. Arthritis Rheum 2005;53(5): 697–702.

27. Ad Hoc Committee on Systemic Lupus Erythematosus Response Criteria for Fatigue. Measurement of fatigue in systemic lupus erythematosus: a systematic review. Arthritis Rheum 2007;57(8):1348–57.

28. Turan Y, Duruoz MT, Bal S, et al. Assessment of fatigue in patients with ankylosing spondylitis. Rheumatol Int 2007;27(9):847–52.

29. Francis K, Bach JR, DeLisa JA. Evaluation and rehabilitation of patients with adult motor neuron disease. Arch Phys Med Rehabil 1999;80(8):951–63.

30. Kos D, Kerckhofs E, Nagels G, et al. Origin of fatigue in multiple sclerosis: review of the literature. Neurorehabil Neural Repair 2008;22(1):91–100.

31. Chipchase SY, Lincoln NB, Radford KA. Measuring fatigue in people with multiple sclerosis. Disabil Rehabil 2003;25(14):778–84.

32. De Groot MH, Phillips SJ, Eskes GA. Fatigue associated with stroke and other neurologic conditions: implications for stroke rehabilitation. Arch Phys Med Rehabil 2003;84(11):1714–20.

33. Kittiwatanapaisan W, Gauthier DK, Williams AM, et al. Fatigue in Myasthenia Gravis patients. J Neurosci Nurs 2003;35(2):87–93, 106.
34. American Psychiatric Association. Diagnostic and statistical manual of mental disorders. Washington, DC: American Psychiatric Association; 2000.
35. Demyttenaere K, De Fruyt J, Stahl SM. The many faces of fatigue in major depressive disorder. Int J Neuropsychopharmacol 2005;8(1):93–105.
36. Belanger L, Ladouceur R, Morin CM. Generalized anxiety disorder and health care use. Can Fam Physician 2005;51:1362–3.
37. Kranzler HR, Manu P, Hesselbrock VM, et al. Substance use disorders in patients with chronic fatigue. Hosp Community Psychiatry 1991;42(9):924–8.
38. Kalkman JS, Schillings ML, van der Werf SP, et al. Experienced fatigue in facioscapulohumeral dystrophy, myotonic dystrophy, and HMSN-I. J Neurol Neurosurg Psychiatr 2005;76(10):1406–9.
39. Wolfe F, Smythe HA, Yunus MB, et al. The American College of Rheumatology 1990 Criteria for the Classification of Fibromyalgia. Report of the Multicenter Criteria Committee. Arthritis Rheum 1990;33(2):160–72.
40. Zijlstra TR, Taal E, van de Laar MA, et al. Validation of a Dutch translation of the fibromyalgia impact questionnaire. Rheumatology (Oxford) 2007;46(1):131–4.
41. Bae SC, Lee JH. Cross-cultural adaptation and validation of the Korean fibromyalgia impact questionnaire in women patients with fibromyalgia for clinical research. Qual Life Res 2004;13(4):857–61.
42. Ericsson A, Mannerkorpi K. Assessment of fatigue in patients with fibromyalgia and chronic widespread pain. Reliability and validity of the Swedish version of the MFI-20. Disabil Rehabil 2007;29(22):1665–70.
43. Garcia-Campayo J, Pascual A, Alda M, et al. The Spanish version of the FibroFatigue Scale: validation of a questionnaire for the observer's assessment of fibromyalgia and chronic fatigue syndrome. Gen Hosp Psychiatry 2006;28(2):154–60.
44. De Vries J, Michielsen H, Van Heck GL, et al. Measuring fatigue in sarcoidosis: the Fatigue Assessment Scale (FAS). Br J Health Psychol 2004;9(Pt 3):279–91.
45. Breslin E, van der Schans C, Breukink S, et al. Perception of fatigue and quality of life in patients with COPD. Chest 1998;114(4):958–64.
46. Schunemann HJ, Puhan M, Goldstein R, et al. Measurement properties and interpretability of the chronic respiratory disease questionnaire (CRQ). COPD 2005; 2(1):81–9.
47. Lichstein KL, Means MK, Noe SL, et al. Fatigue and sleep disorders. Behav Res Ther 1997;35(8):733–40.
48. Barnes EA, Bruera E. Fatigue in patients with advanced cancer: a review. Int J Gynecol Cancer 2002;12(5):424–8.
49. Mitchell SA, Berger AM. Cancer-related fatigue: the evidence base for assessment and management. Cancer J 2006;12(5):374–87.
50. Stasi R, Abriani L, Beccaglia P, et al. Cancer-related fatigue: evolving concepts in evaluation and treatment. Cancer 2003;98(9):1786–801.
51. Jacobsen PB. Assessment of fatigue in cancer patients. J Natl Cancer Inst Monogr 2004;(32):93–7.
52. Jean-Pierre P, Figueroa-Moseley CD, Kohli S, et al. Assessment of cancer-related fatigue: implications for clinical diagnosis and treatment. Oncologist 2007; 12(Suppl 1):11–21.
53. Richardson A. Measuring fatigue in patients with cancer. Support Care Cancer 1998;6(2):94–100.
54. Fisk JD, Doble SE. Construction and validation of a fatigue impact scale for daily administration (D-FIS). Qual Life Res 2002;11(3):263–72.

55. Schwartz JE, Jandorf L, Krupp LB. The measurement of fatigue: a new instrument. J Psychosom Res 1993;37(7):753–62.
56. Huet PM, Deslauriers J, Tran A, et al. Impact of fatigue on the quality of life of patients with primary biliary cirrhosis. Am J Gastroenterol 2000;95(3):760–7.
57. Bjornsson E, Simren M, Olsson R, et al. Fatigue in patients with primary sclerosing cholangitis. Scand J Gastroenterol 2004;39(10):961–8.
58. Dwight MM, Kowdley KV, Russo JE, et al. Depression, fatigue, and functional disability in patients with chronic hepatitis C. J Psychosom Res 2000;49(5):311–7.
59. Bonner A, Wellard S, Caltabiano M. Levels of fatigue in people with ESRD living in far North Queensland. J Clin Nurs 2008;17(1):90–8.
60. Jhamb M, Weisbord SD, Steel JL, et al. Fatigue in patients receiving maintenance dialysis: a review of definitions, measures, and contributing factors. Am J Kidney Dis 2008;52(2):353–65.
61. Lovas K, Loge JH, Husebye ES. Subjective health status in Norwegian patients with Addison's disease. Clin Endocrinol (Oxf) 2002;56(5):581–8.
62. Smith OR, Michielsen HJ, Pelle AJ, et al. Symptoms of fatigue in chronic heart failure patients: clinical and psychological predictors. Eur J Heart Fail 2007; 9(9):922–7.
63. Mota DD, Pimenta CA. Self-report instruments for fatigue assessment: a systematic review. Res Theory Nurs Pract 2006;20(1):49–78.
64. Belmont A, Agar N, Hugeron C, et al. Fatigue and traumatic brain injury. Ann Readapt Med Phys 2006;49(6):283–8, 370–4.

Functional Neuroimaging of Fatigue

John DeLuca, PhD, ABPP[a,b,c,]*, Helen M. Genova, PhD[a],
Emlyn J. Capili, BA[d], Glenn R. Wylie, D Phil[a,b]

KEYWORDS

- Fatigue • Functional neuroimaging
- Basal ganglia • Cognitive • Frontal lobes

Fatigue is one of the most common symptoms observed in numerous medical populations. It has been conceptualized as both a symptom and a syndrome. As a symptom, fatigue has many causes ranging from medical conditions (eg, infections, cancer, thyroid abnormalities, coronary heart disease), insults to the brain (eg, traumatic brain injury [TBI], MS, Parkinson disease [PD], stroke), psychiatric disorders (eg, depression, somatization), medications (eg, antihistamines), and even unhealthy lifestyles. Little is known about the mechanisms that cause fatigue in these conditions. As a syndrome or disease, fatigue has been recognized as the major part of a group of "unexplained" illnesses, such as CFS, neurasthenia, Da Costa syndrome, and so on, in which there is little understanding of its causes.

Fatigue is not always seen as a pathologic feature of a medical condition, as it is also a common problem affecting otherwise healthy individuals. It has been observed as a common problem affecting up to 40% of the population based on community-based samples.[1,2] It is often one of the primary complaints in visits to both primary care physicians and hospitals[3] and can have a significant negative effect on quality of life.[4]

Fatigue is not a unitary concept in terms of both its definition and its measurement. Although the multidimensional nature of fatigue has been recognized for more than 100 years,[5] definitions of fatigue have largely been tied to its subjective nature. For instance, the Multiple Sclerosis Council for Clinical Practice Guidelines[6] defines

[a] Kessler Foundation Research Center, 1199 Pleasant Valley Way, West Orange, NJ 07052, USA
[b] Department of Physical Medicine and Rehabilitation, University of Medicine and Dentistry of New Jersey—New Jersey Medical School, Newark, NJ, USA
[c] Department of Neurology and Neuroscience, University of Medicine and Dentistry of New Jersey—New Jersey Medical School, Newark, NJ, USA
[d] Graduate School of Biomedical Science, University of Medicine and Dentistry of New Jersey—New Jersey Medical School, Newark, NJ, USA
* Corresponding author. Kessler Foundation Research Center, Neuropsychology and Neuroscience Laboratory, 1199 Pleasant Valley Way, West Orange, NJ 07052, USA.
E-mail address: jdeluca@kesslerfoundation.net (J. DeLuca).

Phys Med Rehabil Clin N Am 20 (2009) 325–337
doi:10.1016/j.pmr.2008.12.007
1047-9651/08/$ – see front matter © 2009 Elsevier Inc. All rights reserved.

pmr.theclinics.com

fatigue as "a subjective lack of physical and/or mental energy that is perceived by the individual or caregiver to interfere with usual and desired activities." However, others have conceptualized fatigue through direct behavioral observation, typically viewed as a performance decrement over time (ie, objective performance). Given these 2 most common conceptualizations of fatigue (feeling state vs performance decrement), the most common finding observed in more than 100 years of inquiry is that these 2 metrics of fatigue do not correlate (see DeLuca[7]). In addition, fatigue has also been divided into other components such as central and peripheral fatigue or as cognitive and physical (or motor) fatigue.

The measurement of fatigue only adds to this confusion. A remarkable number of fatigue questionnaires have been developed over the years to assess subjective fatigue. Such inventories range in length from single-item scales (eg, Borg[8]), to multidimensional scales, which claim to assess various dimensions of fatigue (eg, physical vs mental). Most of the items on these scales have a good deal of item similarity and correlate highly with each other, whereas some items claim to be specific to a target audience. One of the major problems, however, with most of the so-called fatigue questionnaires is the construct contamination that mars the validity of such scales. For instance, fatigue inventories often include items on sleepiness and cognition, both of which may not be associated with fatigue (see DeLuca[7] for a review).

In addition to the nebulous qualities of its definition and measurement, the pathophysiology of fatigue remains elusive. A number of pathophysiological mechanisms have been proposed, including immune system dysregulation, impaired nerve conduction, neuroendocrine and neurotransmitter dysregulation, and energy depletion. In addition, a great deal of research has focused on damage to the central nervous system (CNS) as the major contributing factor to fatigue. In particular, research using neuroimaging has begun to provide evidence that several distinct areas of the CNS may be specifically involved in fatigue.

While traditional magnetic resonance imaging (MRI) provides images of brain structure, functional imaging techniques such as functional MRI (fMRI) and positron emission tomography (PET) are techniques that assess functional changes in the brain. fMRI primarily uses the blood oxygen level-dependent (BOLD) contrast as an index of neuronal activity. PET measures glucose metabolism with the aid of radioactive tracers.

The major thrust of this article is on what we are beginning to learn about fatigue from studies using functional neuroimaging; though, for completeness, we begin with a brief review of the structural imaging studies.

A search of the functional imaging literature on fatigue yielded studies almost exclusively with 2 populations: MS and CFS (**Fig. 1**). Therefore, the primary focus of this article is to review the existing neuroimaging research on fatigue in MS and CFS.

FATIGUE IN MS

Fatigue is one of the most common symptoms reported by patients with MS.[9] It frequently presents as the primary symptom at the time of diagnosis, and patients often report fatigue as the most troubling feature of the disease.[9] Fatigue has been shown to be significantly associated with reduced activities of daily living,[10] and it negatively affects employment and social relationships in persons with MS.[9,11] Fatigue in MS tends to be associated more with affect state than with both measures of disease activity (eg, EDSS) and other neurologic metrics (eg, neuroimaging).[9]

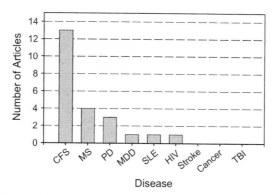

Fig. 1. Number of functional neuroimaging articles published by clinical group. CFS, chronic fatigue syndrome; HIV, human immunodeficiency virus; MDD, major depressive disorder; MS, multiple sclerosis; PD, Parkinson disease; SLE, systemic lupus erythematosus; TBI, traumatic brain injury. Reviews and case studies were excluded. For each disease, we initially searched the PubMed database with the terms "("magnetic resonance imaging" OR MRI) OR ("diffusion tensor imaging" OR DTI) OR ("magnetic resonance spectroscopy" OR MRS) OR ("positron emission tomography" OR PET) OR ("single photon emission computerized tomography" OR SPECT) OR (magnetoencephalography OR MEG) OR ("magnetic resonance" OR MR) OR ("functional magnetic resonance imaging" OR fMRI) OR neuroimaging," then within those results, we searched for "fatigue," and then within those results, we searched for each of the disease types.

Fatigue in MS Using Structural MRI Studies

A number of studies have been conducted during the past 10 years examining the relationship between self-reported measures of fatigue and structural damage in MS using MRI. Most of these studies focused on using self-report of fatigue in groups of fatigued and nonfatigued MS participants and measured cerebral abnormalities, usually T2- and T1-weighted total lesion load in discrete cerebral areas and/or cerebral atrophy. The earlier studies conducted found no significant relationship between these indices of pathology and self-reported fatigue.[12–16] To illustrate, Mainero and colleagues[17] associated increased fatigue with disruption of the blood–brain barrier, which would allow cytokines to infiltrate the CNS. They hypothesized that the presence of gadolinium-enhancing (Gd+) lesions on MRI scans would be indicative of this blood–brain barrier disruption. Yet no relationship was found between the number and volume of Gd-enhancing lesions and fatigue severity at any time point studied.

Although most studies using MRI have not found a relationship between structural indices and fatigue, a few studies have reported positive results.[18,19] For example, Marrie and colleagues (2005)[20] used a longitudinal design to examine the relationship between brain atrophy changes and subjective fatigue during 8 years. Although no relationship between pathology and fatigue was observed after 2 years, a significant change was observed in fatigue effect during the 8-year period. This relationship was maintained after adjusting for disability, mood, and the subjects' baseline MRI.

More advanced MRI techniques, such as diffusion tensor imaging (DTI) and magnetization transfer, have also failed to show a significant relationship with self-reported fatigue in persons with MS.[21,22]

Functional Neuroimaging of Fatigue in MS

The most common functional imaging techniques to study fatigue in MS are PET and fMRI. Roelcke and colleagues[23] used 18F-fluorodeoxyglucose PET (FDG-PET) to measure cerebral glucose metabolism in 47 participants with MS. Compared with MS subjects without fatigue, the fatigued MS group showed significant hypometabolism in the putamen, prefrontal and premotor cortex, and the right supplementary motor area. The Fatigue Severity Scale (FSS) scores were negatively correlated with glucose uptake in the right prefrontal cortex (PFC). Hypometabolism in the fatigued MS group extended from the rostral putamen toward the lateral head of the caudate nucleus. In contrast, the fatigued MS group showed elevated glucose metabolism in the anterior cingulate and the cerebellar vermis. The authors concluded that dysfunctional cerebral activity in both the basal ganglia and prefrontal regions is responsible for fatigue in persons with MS.

The primary technique employed to examine functional cerebral activity of fatigue in persons with MS is fMRI. Fillipi and colleagues[16] divided their MS sample into fatigued and nonfatigued groups based on the FSS and measured BOLD activation during performance of a motor task. They reported that the MS group with fatigue had significantly less functional cerebral activation in several regions involved in motor planning and execution compared with that in the MS group without fatigue. These regions included the ipsilateral precuneus, ipsilateral cerebellar hemispheres, contralateral middle frontal gyrus, and contralateral thalamus. A negative correlation between the FSS score and cerebral activation in the contralateral thalamus was also observed. The thalamus is known to be a major relay station between motor and prefrontal regions and basal ganglia. Filipi and colleagues[16] hypothesized that these findings suggested a disruption of cortical–subcortical circuits associated with functional activity between the thalamus, basal ganglia, and motor and prefrontal regions of the frontal lobes. Although most regions of the brain showed hypoactivity, the fatigued MS group did show increased activation in the anterior cingulate relative to that in the nonfatigued MS group. The authors suggested that anterior cingulate recruitment in the fatigued group may represent a "compensatory mechanism" because of the increased effort required to perform the task. These authors also conducted an analysis of structural MRI lesions and found no significant differences in lesion load quantity between the fatigued and nonfatigued MS groups. Taken together, such data suggest that functional cerebral changes in the brain may be more sensitive than structural imaging in identifying the cerebral underpinnings associated with fatigue in persons with MS.

All of the studies reviewed thus far have used subjective report as the measure of fatigue in fMRI studies. A more recent approach is to assess fatigue objectively, by inducing cognitive fatigue during fMRI acquisition and examining the brain regions associated with such fatigue. Successful attempts at objective measurement of cognitive fatigue have focused on decreased behavioral performance in tasks requiring *sustained mental effort.*[7] This approach is similar to that typically thought of in the motor fatigue literature, where fatigue has been defined as a failure to maintain a required force or output of power during sustained or repeated muscle contraction. There is indeed considerable support for such an objective assessment of cognitive fatigue in clinical populations (see DeLuca,[7] for a review). Two recent studies used this design of objectively measuring cognitive fatigue during fMRI acquisition in persons with MS.

DeLuca and colleagues[24] attempted to induce cognitive fatigue in persons with MS and in healthy controls (HCs) by administering 4 trials of a sustained attention task ie, modified Symbol Digit Modalities Task or (mSDMT) during fMRI acquisition. It was hypothesized that participants with MS would show a greater *increase* in cerebral activity while performing the mSDMT across time compared with that in HCs. Importantly, based on the various studies in HCs, DeLuca and colleagues[24] hypothesized observing a *decrease* in cerebral activation to repeated administration of the mSDMT tasks over time in healthy individuals (eg, Petersen and colleagues;[25] Raichle and colleagues;[26] Koch and colleagues[27]). That is, DeLuca and colleagues[24] operationally defined "cognitive fatigue" as an increase in cerebral activation across the 4 trials of a processing-speed task in individuals with MS, relative to that in the control group, which would exhibit a decrease in brain activity across time. DeLuca and colleagues[24] found no group differences in performance accuracy across the 4 trials of the cognitive task. The MS group showed increased cerebral activation in key areas of the brain compared with that in the healthy group, which showed decreased activation (**Fig. 2**). These regions included the precuneus, superior parietal lobe (BA 7), medial/orbital frontal gyrus, inferior parietal lobe, and the caudate in the basal ganglia. One limitation of the DeLuca and colleagues[24] study was that subjective fatigue was not assessed, so it was unclear how these results would change if differing levels of subjective fatigue were taken into account.

What was particularly important about the DeLuca and colleagues[24] study was that it was specifically designed to test the current model of brain mechanisms responsible for central fatigue proposed by Chaudhuri and Behan.[28,29] Chaudhuri and Behan hypothesize that "central fatigue" is a function of the nonmotor function of the basal ganglia. These authors suggest that "alterations in the normal flow of

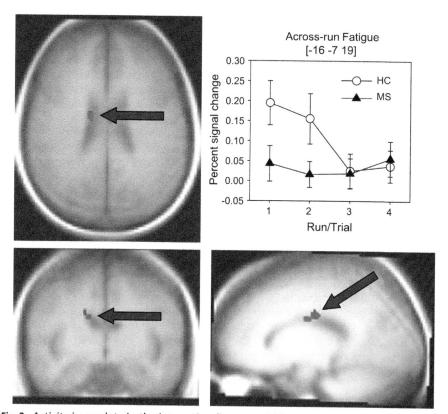

Fig. 2. Activity in caudate in the interaction (inset graph) between groups. (*Reprinted from Journal of the Neurological Sciences*, 270(1–2), DeLuca, J, Genova, HM, Hillary, FG, Wylie, G, Neural correlates of cognitive fatigue in multiple sclerosis using functional MRI, 28–39, Copyright (2008); with permission from Elsevier.)

sequential activation within the basal ganglia system affecting the neural integrator and the cortical feedback by the associated loop of the striato-thalamo-cortical fibers is a possible mechanism of central fatigue …" (p40). The findings of the DeLuca and colleagues[24] study of altered cerebral activation within the basal ganglia and frontal lobes during cognitive fatigue lend direct support to the Chaudhuri and Behan[28,29] model.

A second study was recently published using objective behavioral performance to measure fatigue in persons with MS using fMRI. Tartaglia and colleagues[30] hypothesized that induced cognitive fatigue could alter cerebral activation patterns associated with motor performance. Specifically, they hypothesized that fatigue experienced by individuals with MS may be related to "greater demands being placed on diminishing functional neural circuits, resulting in reduced capacity to respond to new demands." Tartaglia and colleagues[30] examined BOLD activation during an experiment that had 3 stages. First, subjects performed a motor task (stage 1); then they performed a challenging cognitive task (the paced auditory serial addition test PASAT; stage 2); finally, they performed the motor task again (stage 3). The HC group showed no significant difference in cerebral activation during the motor task when the motor task in stage 1 was compared with the same task in stage 3 (ie, pre- vs post-PASAT). The MS group, however, showed increased activity in multiple regions after performance of the PASAT (that is, when the motor task in stage 3 was compared with the same task in stage 1). These included the bilateral cingulate gyrus, the post-central gyrus, and the right PFC. In fact, although the HCs showed decreased activation in the motor task after PASAT performance (ie, stage 3 vs stage 1), in the MS group the activation in all recruited areas was increased. The authors concluded that induced cognitive fatigue could alter brain activation in an unrelated motor task, resulting in increased cerebral activity in persons with MS. One limitation of the study is the absence of a nonfatigued MS group, making it difficult to determine whether these findings were truly due to fatigue or to some other disease-related process.

In summary, studies using structural MRI have yielded mixed results at best in identifying the underlying cerebral structures associated with fatigue in MS. Functional imaging, particularly fMRI, has been much more successful. Although most studies have used subjective report as the primary index of fatigue, a few have measured fatigue using objective performance during the imaging session.

CHRONIC FATIGUE SYNDROME

CFS is a heterogeneous illness characterized primarily by severe and debilitating fatigue as well as infectious, rheumatologic, and neuropsychiatric symptoms.[31] A number of structural and functional imaging studies have been conducted on individuals with CFS. Given that fatigue is the defining characteristic of CFS, one could expect that the neuroimaging studies conducted would reveal much about fatigue itself. However, it should be recognized that some of the differences in brain structure and function between individuals with CFS and HCs might not be related to fatigue but to differences in subject characteristics (eg, psychopathology). Thus, one should be cautious in attributing group differences in functional imaging to effects of fatigue based on simple comparisons between individuals with CFS and HCs. Only studies that measure fatigue and use this measurement in the imaging data can be used to make inferences about brain mechanisms involved in fatigue in CFS. Unfortunately, only a handful of recent studies have employed this approach in CFS. Most of the imaging studies have simply compared brain structure or function in patients with CFS to those without CFS and assumed that the differences are related to fatigue.

Structural Neuroimaging in CFS

The early studies in CFS focused primarily on structural imaging. Although several early studies showed an increased number of white matter hyperintensities on MRI in CFS versus HCs (eg, Buchwald and colleagues;[32] Natelson and colleagues[33]), several other studies did not (eg, Schwartz and colleagues;[34] Cope and colleagues[35]). Lange and colleagues[36] found significantly more subcortical white matter hyperintensities in a group of CFS subjects without psychiatric illness (concurrent or historic) compared with those in the CFS group with concurrent psychiatric illness. A similar pattern of results was reported by Greco and colleagues.[37]

Cook and colleagues[38] divided individuals with CFS into those with cerebral abnormalities and those without and found that CFS participants with cerebral abnormalities reported more impairments in physical functioning on the short-form 36-item health survey than those of CFS subjects without cerebral abnormalities. Measuring cerebral volume using MRI, Lange and colleagues[39] found that CFS participants had larger lateral ventricle volumes compared with those of HCs. Okada and colleagues[40] reported significantly reduced gray matter volume in prefrontal areas, bilaterally in their CFS group. Gray matter volume in the right PFC was correlated with the severity of self-reported fatigue, suggesting a prominent role of the PFC in the phenomenology of fatigue. De Lange and colleagues[41] have reported that this reduction in gray matter volume can be partially reversed by cognitive-behavioral therapy.

Functional Neuroimaging in CFS

Using single photon emission computerized tomography (SPECT), Schwartz and colleagues[34] found increased perfusion in the lateral frontal cortex and lateral and medial temporal cortex in their CFS group. Increased perfusion using SPECT in CFS has also been observed in the right thalamus and basal ganglia (pallidum and putamen).[42] Costa and colleagues,[43] however, reported decreases in perfusion in the brainstem of their CFS sample using SPECT. Although these studies showing systemic differences in blood flow are of interest, their role in fatigue is unclear. In contrast, Fischler and colleagues[44] examined whether there was a relationship between cerebral perfusion using SPECT and physical or mental fatigue in persons with CFS. No relationship between fatigue and cerebral perfusion was found.

A few studies in CFS using PET have been published. Using 18-FDG-PET, CFS subjects showed decreases in cerebral metabolism in the frontal lobes.[45] Siessmeier and colleagues[46] reported abnormalities in the anterior cingulate gyrus/mesial frontal cortex and orbital frontal cortex in about half of their CFS sample. However, no significant relationships were found between reductions in glucose metabolism and fatigue in CFS.

Another approach has been to use a challenging task that one might expect would induce fatigue and to investigate the pattern of activity during performance of this task in individuals with CFS relative to that in HCs. This approach has shown CFS to be associated with more widespread and diffuse regional cerebral blood flow in frontal, temporal, and thalamic regions relative to that in controls[47] using SPECT. Using fMRI, Lange and colleagues[48] used a challenging cognitive task and found that persons with CFS showed more diffuse and bilateral activity than that of HCs. Although HCs showed left-lateralized activity in frontal and parietal regions, individuals with CFS showed bilateral activity in frontal and parietal regions (see also Lange and colleagues[49]). Other work has underscored the importance of the right prefrontal areas, showing that as the difficulty of a working memory task increased, these areas are recruited.[50] All of these studies that used challenging tasks as the experimental paradigm show group differences between individuals with CFS and controls. However, it is unclear whether these differences have anything to do with fatigue itself, as no specific relationship with measures of fatigue was made.

More recent studies in CFS have begun to explicitly include measures of fatigue in the analysis of functional imaging data. Cook and colleagues[51] demonstrated a relationship between subjective fatigue and functional brain activity using fMRI while performing a cognitive task (modified PASAT) in persons with CFS. They found that subjective reports of fatigue after task performance correlated positively with brain activity in several areas including the cerebellum (vermis), the cingulate region (middle and posterior), inferior frontal gyrus, superior temporal gyrus, parietal regions, and the hippocampus. Tanaka and colleagues[52] used a similar approach but looked at brain activity associated both with a difficult, fatiguing, visual search task and activity associated with a completely extraneous, task-irrelevant change in auditory stimulation using fMRI. The functional activity associated with the search task did not differ significantly between the CFS and control groups nor did it correlate with subjective ratings of fatigue. However, the CFS group showed significantly less cerebral activity than that of the HC group during the task-irrelevant change in auditory stimulation, and the activity was correlated with subjective ratings of fatigue. The authors suggested that CFS subjects may have less processing "capacity" and, therefore, have less ability to process task-irrelevant stimuli than that of HCs.

A novel approach to the study of fatigue in persons with CFS was adopted by Caseras and colleagues,[53] who analyzed the BOLD response recorded while persons with CFS were watching either a fatigue-inducing scenario (video clip) or an anxiety-inducing scenario. Following each scenario, subjects rated their feelings of fatigue and anxiety. Results showed that the fatiguing clips induced greater feelings of fatigue than the anxiety-clips in both the CFS and HC groups ($P<.001$) and that the CFS group was more fatigued than the control group ($P<.001$). Moreover, when watching the fatiguing clips, the CFS group showed increased activity in the cerebellum and occipito-parietal regions bilaterally extending toward the cingulate gyrus, the left hippocampal gyrus, and the left caudate nucleus. For the HC group, increased activity was seen in the right dorsolateral and bilateral medial PFC (extending toward the anterior cingulate), right insula, and right caudate nucleus when watching the fatiguing clips than the anxiety-inducing clips. Importantly, fatigue was associated with activity in the basal ganglia (caudate) for both the CFS and HC groups. In addition, the CFS group showed more activation in the posterior regions and those associated with emotion (cingulate), whereas the HC group showed more activity in the frontal regions associated with executive control. Lastly, the regions activated in the CFS group in the Caseras and colleagues[53] study showed broad overlap with those reported by Cook and colleagues,[51] even though the 2 studies used widely different paradigms and analyses.

In summary, although there is evidence for structural changes in the brain for persons with CFS, including white matter damage and gray matter volume, it is unclear how these changes are associated with fatigue per se. Functional neuroimaging studies appear to offer greater promise in understanding the cerebral mechanisms of fatigue in CFS, although caution is needed in interpreting functional imaging studies that just display group difference, as these characteristics may not be directly related to fatigue. When fatigue is specifically assessed and related to functional brain activity, areas that appear to be significantly associated with fatigue include the basal ganglia, the cingulate, the cerebellum, and the parietal cortex. Interestingly, some of these structures, particularly the basal ganglia, support the Chaudhuri and Behan,[28,29] model of fatigue. It is likely that further investigation of this set of brain regions may prove fruitful in our understanding of fatigue in CFS.

Functional neuroimaging in other clinical populations

As illustrated in **Fig. 1**, there are only about a handful of studies examining the association between subjectively reported fatigue and neurocognitive measures in several other clinical populations, including systemic lupus erythematosus (SLE), major depressive disorder (MDD), Parkinson disease (PD), and TBI. Overall, these studies have shown mixed results. For example, when a correlation was sought between fatigue (using the FSS) and cerebral blood flow (CBF) in SLE (using SPECT), no brain region showed such a correlation.[54] This was found despite the fact that subjects with SLE showed reliable disturbances in CBF compared with those of controls. No relationship between subjective fatigue and FDG-PET abnormalities was observed in a small sample of persons who were human immunodeficiency virus (HIV) positive.[55] However, in MDD, fatigue was found to covary with measures of functional brain activity in 1 study. Brody and colleagues[56] examined the association between change in depressive symptoms and change in regional brain metabolism using PET from before to after treatment. Decreases in fatigue from pre- to post-treatment correlated with decreases in ventral PFC activity (metabolism) bilaterally. That is, as fatigue lessened (improved), there was less activity in ventral PFC. This is a promising finding but must be interpreted with caution, since a fairly liberal activation threshold was used ($P<.05$, not corrected for multiple comparisons).

In PD, 2 studies have looked at the availability of dopamine in the basal ganglia, using SPECT.[57,58] Schifitto and colleagues[57] compared fatigued PD subjects to non-fatigued patients and found that though fatigued patients had significantly more neurologic impairment (as measured by each subset of the Unified Parkinson Disease Rating Scale and Hoehn-Yayr scale), there was no difference in their measure of striatal dopamine transporter density, $[^{123}I]$-β-CIT SPECT in the striatum, caudate, or putamen. Weintraub and colleagues[58] found a trend for a correlation ($P = .11$) between their measure of fatigue in PD subjects (the profile of mood states) and the distribution of striatal dopamine transporter in the left anterior putamen. Although this association was clearly not significant, the cohort of PD patients in this study were not reliably more fatigued than the HC group, suggesting that perhaps more robust effects would be found with more fatigued participants. Finally, Abe and colleagues[59] investigated the correlation between cerebral perfusion, using SPECT, and fatigue (using the FSS) in PD subjects. These researchers found a significant correlation between FSS and perfusion in the frontal lobes such that more fatigue (higher FSS scores) was associated with less frontal perfusion.

Using a similar paradigm to that employed by DeLuca and colleagues[24] in their fMRI study of fatigue in MS, Kohl and colleagues[60] measured cognitive fatigue objectively during fMRI in persons with TBI. Briefly, a cognitive task requiring sustained attention (ie, SDMT) was administered 3 times for blocks (or "runs") lasting approximately 5 minutes during fMRI acquisition for both TBI and HC subjects. Based on the logic of the DeLuca and colleagues[24] study in MS (see also above), Kohl and colleagues[60] hypothesized that TBI participants would show an *increase* in cerebral activity on the mSDMT in areas of the brain hypothesized to be associated with fatigue, whereas HCs would show *decreased* activation. That is, Kohl and colleagues[60] operationally defined "cognitive fatigue" in 2 ways: an increase in cerebral activation from the first half to the second half of the 3 runs of the processing-speed task in individuals with TBI compared with that in HCs (within-run fatigue) and an increase in cerebral activation across the 3 runs of the processing-speed task (across-run fatigue). Behaviorally, no significant difference in performance accuracy was observed between the TBI and HC group, although the TBI was significantly slower in performing the task. However, in the fMRI data, effects consistent with within-run fatigue were found in the middle frontal gyrus (BA 10), the superior parietal lobe (BA 7), and the basal ganglia (the putamen). Effects consistent with across-run fatigue were also seen and were confined to the anterior cingulate (BA 32). These data were interpreted as supporting the Chaudhuri and Behan[28,29] model of central fatigue.

SUMMARY

Clearly, the use of functional neuroimaging for the study of fatigue is in its infancy. Relatively few studies focusing on fatigue using functional neuroimaging techniques have been published, and the few that exist focus primarily on persons with MS and CFS. The vast majority of these studies have examined self-reported fatigue, an approach that benefits from ease of administration but suffers from significant difficulties in interpretation. For example, we know that self-reported fatigue most often correlates with the degree of psychopathology.[1] We also know that with more than 100 years of inquiry, self-reported fatigue does *not* correlate with objective measures of fatigue.[5,7] As such, when functional imaging studies show a relationship between self-reported fatigue and activities in distinct areas of the brain, one must remain cautious about the interpretation of these results. A more recent approach in the functional imaging literature is to assess fatigue behaviorally during scanning and relate such objective measures of fatigue with cerebral activation. Although this is a new and novel approach, it remains unclear if this approach of operationally defining fatigue behaviorally will be a more valid paradigm in understanding the elusive construct of fatigue.

Although fatigue is extraordinarily common as a symptom in many neurologic and psychiatric diseases, little is known about its precise mechanism. Chaudhuri and Behan[28,29] hypothesized that the nonmotor functions of the basal ganglia play a key role in central fatigue. Specifically, they posit that fatigue is due to "alterations in the normal flow of sequential activation within the basal ganglia system affecting the neural integrator and the cortical feedback by the associated loop of the striato-thalamo-cortical fibers is a possible mechanism of central fatigue ..." (p40). Therefore, other regions interacting with the basal ganglia may also contribute to fatigue, including the frontal cortex, thalamus, and the amygdala. In general, the functional imaging studies reviewed in this article tend to generally support the suggestion that damage to cortical–subcortical circuitry might be to blame for fatigue as well.[14,16,23,61,62] If indeed fatigue is associated with functional impairment in a cortical–subcortical circuitry, it might be that studies that have examined structural damage (eg, total lesion load throughout the brain) may simply not provide the sensitivity required to detect a relationship between fatigue and pathology.

After more than 100 years of frustration, it appears that functional neuroimaging techniques promise to provide an exciting potential for significant advances in our elusive understanding of the brain mechanisms associated with fatigue in clinical populations.

REFERENCES

1. Wessely S, Hotopf M, Sharpe D. Chronic fatigue and its syndromes. New York: Oxford University Press; 1998.
2. Lewis G, Wessely S. The epidemiology of fatigue: more questions than answers. J Epidemiol Community Health 1992;46(2):92–7.
3. Manu P, Lane T, Matthews D. Chronic fatigue syndromes in clinical practice. Psychother Psychosom 1992;58(2):60–8.

4. Nelson E, Kirk J, McHugo G, et al. Chief complaint fatigue: a longitudinal study from the patient's perspective. Fam Pract Res J 1987;6(4):175–88.
5. Mosso A. Fatigue. London: Swan Sonnenschein and Co; 1904.
6. Paralyzed Veterans of America. Fatigue and multiple sclerosis: evidenced-based management strategies for fatigue in multiple sclerosis. Washington (DC): Multiple Sclerosis Council for Clinical Practice Guidelines; 1998.
7. DeLuca J. Fatigue: its definition, its study and its future. In: DeLuca J, editor. Fatigue as a window to the brain. Cambridge (MA): MIT Press; 2005. p. 319–25.
8. Borg G. Perceived exertion as an indicator of somatic stress. J Rehabil Med 1970; 2(2):92–8.
9. Krupp L, Christodoulou C, Schombert H. Multiple sclerosis and fatigue. In: DeLuca J, editor. Fatigue as a window to the brain. Cambridge (MA): MIT Press; 2005. p. 61–71.
10. Barak Y, Achiron A. Cognitive fatigue in multiple sclerosis: findings from a two-wave screening project. J Neurol Sci 2006;245(1–2):73–6.
11. Skerrett T, Moss-Morris R. Fatigue and social impairment in multiple sclerosis: the role of patients' cognitive and behavioral responses to their symptoms. J Psychosom Res 2006;61(5):587–93.
12. van der Werf S, Jongen P, Lycklama à Nijeholt G, et al. Fatigue in multiple sclerosis: interrelations between fatigue complaints, cerebral MRI abnormalities and neurological disability. J Neurol Sci 1998;160(2):164–70.
13. Bakshi R, Miletich R, Henschel K, et al. Fatigue in multiple sclerosis: cross-sectional correlation with brain MRI findings in 71 patients. Neurology 1999;53(5):1151–3.
14. Tartaglia M, Narayanan S, Francis S, et al. The relationship between diffuse axonal damage and fatigue in multiple sclerosis. Arch Neurol 2004;61(2):201–7.
15. Téllez N, Alonso J, Río J, et al. The basal ganglia: a substrate for fatigue in multiple sclerosis. Neuroradiology 2008;50(1):17–23.
16. Filippi M, Rocca M, Colombo B, et al. Functional magnetic resonance imaging correlates of fatigue in multiple sclerosis. Neuroimage 2002;15(3):559–67.
17. Mainero C, Faroni J, Gasperini C, et al. Fatigue and magnetic resonance imaging activity in multiple sclerosis. J Neurol 1999;246(6):454–8.
18. Colombo B, Martinelli Boneschi F, Rossi P, et al. MRI and motor evoked potential findings in nondisabled multiple sclerosis patients with and without symptoms of fatigue. J Neurol 2000;247(7):506–9.
19. Tedeschi G, Dinacci D, Lavorgna L, et al. Correlation between fatigue and brain atrophy and lesion load in multiple sclerosis patients independent of disability. J Neurol Sci 2007;263(1–2):15–9.
20. Marrie R, Fisher E, Miller D, et al. Association of fatigue and brain atrophy in multiple sclerosis. J Neurol Sci 2005;228(2):161–6.
21. Codella M, Rocca M, Colombo B, et al. Cerebral grey matter pathology and fatigue in patients with multiple sclerosis: a preliminary study. J Neurol Sci 2002a;194(1):71–4.
22. Codella M, Rocca M, Colombo B, et al. A preliminary study of magnetization transfer and diffusion tensor MRI of multiple sclerosis patients with fatigue. J Neurol 2002b;249(5):535–7.
23. Roelcke U, Kappos L, Lechner-Scott J, et al. Reduced glucose metabolism in the frontal cortex and basal ganglia of multiple sclerosis patients with fatigue: a 18F-fluorodeoxyglucose positron emission tomography study. Neurology 1997;48(6):1566–71.
24. DeLuca J, Genova H, Hillary F, et al. Neural correlates of cognitive fatigue in multiple sclerosis using functional MRI. J Neurol Sci 2008;270(1–2):28–39.

25. Petersen S, van Mier H, Fiez J, et al. The effects of practice on the functional anatomy of task performance. Proc Natl Acad Sci U S A 1998;95(3):853–60.

26. Raichle M, Fiez J, Videen T, et al. Practice-related changes in human brain functional anatomy during nonmotor learning. Cereb Cortex 1994;4(1):8–26.

27. Koch K, Wagner G, von Consbruch K, et al. Temporal changes in neural activation during practice of information retrieval from short-term memory: an fMRI study. Brain Res 2006;1107:140–50.

28. Chaudhuri A, Behan P. Fatigue and basal ganglia. J Neurol Sci 2000;179(Suppl 1–2):34–42.

29. Chaudhuri A, Behan P. Fatigue in neurological populations. Lancet 2004;363: 978–88.

30. Tartaglia M, Narayanan S, Arnold D. Mental fatigue alters the pattern and increases the volume of cerebral activation required for a motor task in multiple sclerosis patients with fatigue. Eur J Neurol 2008;15(4):413–9.

31. Fukuda K, Straus SE, Hickie I, et al. The chronic fatigue syndrome: a comprehensive approach to its definition and study. Ann Intern Med 1994;121:953–9.

32. Buchwald D, Cheney P, Peterson D, et al. A chronic illness characterized by fatigue, neurologic and immunologic disorders, and active human herpes virus type 6 infection. Ann Intern Med 1992;116(2):103–13.

33. Natelson B, Cohen J, Brassloff I, et al. A controlled study of brain magnetic resonance imaging in patients with the chronic fatigue syndrome. J Neurol Sci 1993; 120(2):213–7.

34. Schwartz R, Garada B, Komaroff A, et al. Detection of intracranial abnormalities in patients with chronic fatigue syndrome: comparison of MR imaging and SPECT. AJR Am J Roentgenol 1994;162(4):935–41.

35. Cope H, Pernet A, Kendall B, et al. Cognitive functioning and magnetic resonance imaging in chronic fatigue. Br J Psychiatry 1995;167(1):86–94.

36. Lange G, DeLuca J, Maldjian J, et al. Brain MRI abnormalities exist in a subset of patients with chronic fatigue syndrome. J Neurol Sci 1999;171(1):3–7.

37. Greco A, Tannock C, Brostoff J, et al. Brain MR in chronic fatigue syndrome. AJNR Am J Neuroradiol 1997;18(7):1265–9.

38. Cook D, Lange G, DeLuca J, et al. Relationship of brain MRI abnormalities and physical functional status in chronic fatigue syndrome. Int J Neurosci 2001; 107(1–2):1–6.

39. Lange G, Holodny A, DeLuca J, et al. Quantitative assessment of cerebral ventricular volumes in chronic fatigue syndrome. Appl Neuropsychol 2001;8(1): 23–30.

40. Okada T, Tanaka M, Kuratsune H, et al. Mechanisms underlying fatigue: a voxel-based morphometric study of chronic fatigue syndrome. BMC Neurol 2004;4(1):4–14.

41. de Lange F, Koers A, Kalkman J, et al. Increase in prefrontal cortical volume following cognitive behavioural therapy in patients with chronic fatigue syndrome. Brain 2008;131(Pt 8):2172–80.

42. MacHale S, Lawrie S, Cavanagh J, et al. Cerebral perfusion in chronic fatigue syndrome and depression. Br J Psychiatry 2000;176:550–6.

43. Costa D, Tannock C, Brostoff J. Brainstem perfusion is impaired in chronic fatigue syndrome. QJM 1995;88(11):767–73.

44. Fischler B, D'Haenen H, Cluydts R, et al. Comparison of 99m Tc HMPAO SPECT scan between chronic fatigue syndrome, major depression and healthy controls: an exploratory study of clinical correlates of regional cerebral blood flow. Neuropsychobiology 1996;34(4):175–83.

45. Tirelli U, Chierichetti F, Tavio M, et al. Brain positron emission tomography (PET) in chronic fatigue syndrome: preliminary data. Am J Med 1998;105(3):54S–8S.
46. Siessmeier T, Nix W, Hardt J, et al. Observer independent analysis of cerebral glucose metabolism in patients with chronic fatigue syndrome. J Neurol Neurosurg Psychiatr 2003;74(7):922–8.
47. Schmaling K, Lewis D, Fiedelak J, et al. Single-photon emission computerized tomography and neurocognitive function in patients with chronic fatigue syndrome. Psychosom Med 2003;65(1):129–36.
48. Lange G, Steffener J, Christodoulou C, et al. FMRI of auditory verbal working memory in severe fatiguing illness. Neuroimage 2000;11(5, Suppl 1):S95.
49. Lange G, Steffener J, Cook D, et al. Objective evidence of cognitive complaints in Chronic Fatigue Syndrome: a BOLD fMRI study of verbal working memory. Neuroimage 2005;26(2):513–24.
50. Caseras X, Mataix-Cols D, Giampietro V, et al. Probing the working memory system in chronic fatigue syndrome: a functional magnetic resonance imaging study using the n-back task. Psychosom Med 2006;68(6):947–55.
51. Cook D, O'Connor P, Lange G, et al. Functional neuroimaging correlates of mental fatigue induced by cognition among chronic fatigue syndrome patients and controls. Neuroimage 2007;36(1):108–22.
52. Tanaka M, Sadato N, Okada T, et al. Reduced responsiveness is an essential feature of chronic fatigue syndrome: a fMRI study. BMC Neurol 2006;6(9) [Epub ahead of print].
53. Caseras X, Mataix-Cols D, Rimes K, et al. The neural correlates of fatigue: an exploratory imaginal fatigue provocation study in chronic fatigue syndrome. Psychol Med 2008;38(7):941–51.
54. Omdal R, Sjöholm H, Koldingsnes W, et al. Fatigue in patients with lupus is not associated with disturbances in cerebral blood flow as detected by SPECT. J Neurol 2005;252:78–83.
55. Andersen AB, Law I, Ostrowski S, et al. Self-reported fatigue common among optimally treated HIV patients: no correlation with cerebral FDG-PET scanning abnormalities. Neuroimmunomodulation 2006;13:69–75.
56. Brody AL, Saxena S, Makdelkern MA, et al. Brain metabolic changes associated with symptom factor improvement in major depressive disorder. Biol Psychiatry 2001;50:171–8.
57. Schifitto G, Friedman JH, Oakes D, et al. Fatigue in levodopa-naive subjects with Parkinson disease. Neurology 2008;71:481–5.
58. Weintraub D, Newberg A, Cary M, et al. Striatal dopamine transporter imaging correlates with anxiety and depression symptoms in Parkinson's disease. J Nucl Med 2005;46(2):227–32.
59. Abe K, Takanashi M, Yanagihara T. Fatigue in patients with Parkinson's disease. Behav Neurol 2000;12:103–6.
60. Kohl AD, Wylie GR, Genova HM, et al. The neural correlates of cognitive fatigue in traumatic brain injury using functional MRI. Brain Injury, in press.
61. Leocani L, Colombo B, Magnani G, et al. Fatigue in multiple sclerosis is associated with abnormal cortical activation to voluntary movement—EEG evidence. Neuroimage 2001;13(6 Pt 1):1186–92.
62. Niepel G, Tench C, Morgan P, et al. Deep gray matter and fatigue in MS: a T1 relaxation time study. J Neurol 2006;253(7):896–902.

Fatigue in Children with Neurologic Impairments

Marykatharine Nutini, DO[a],*, Michelle Karczewski, MD[b],
Jaishree Capoor, MD, FAAP[c]

KEYWORDS

- Chronic fatigue • Children • Adolescents
- Neuromuscular illness • Physiatry • Pediatric rehabilitation

In recent years, medical research has taken a great interest in chronic fatigue affecting adults. Multiple theories as to possible etiologies have been examined, and various treatments have been studied. Despite this, many questions still remain regarding this common but complex phenomenon. It is hoped that further research will guide its management and significantly improve the lives of patients impacted by this disabling illness.

Unfortunately, the focus on adult chronic fatigue overshadows the lack of attention to evaluating this condition in the pediatric population. This deficiency is particularly worrisome, as chronic fatigue in a child would theoretically have different implications when compared with that in an adult. If the child's play and school activities were to be limited secondary to fatigue, the physical, educational, and social development of that child could be delayed. One study reported that these children demonstrated increased absence from school (20-60 days), with subsequent decline in academic performance, reduction in extracurricular activities, and adverse effects on peer relationships.[1]

Although it appears that this oversight is slowly being addressed, more information regarding this subset would prove valuable, as children seem to be affected to a similar extent as adults.[2] The overall prevalence of this underdiagnosed pediatric ailment has been approximated as 1.2% to 1.9%, which is comparable to the prevalence of chronic fatigue in adults.[3] Like adults, those children typically affected are female with a ratio of 2:1 as compared to males.[1,3] They tend to be in their early teenage years

[a] The Mount Sinai Hospital, 1425 Madison Avenue, Box 1240, Department of Rehabilitation Medicine, 4th Floor, New York, NY 10029, USA
[b] NewYork-Presbyterian Hospital, WeillCornell Medical Center, 525 East 68th Street, Department of Rehabilitation Medicine - Baker 16, New York, NY 10065, USA
[c] Elmhurst Hospital/Mount Sinai School of Medicine/Blythedale Children's Hospital, 95 Bradhurst Avenue, Elmhurst, NY 11595, USA
* Corresponding author.
E-mail address: marykaynutini@gmail.com (M. Nutini).

Phys Med Rehabil Clin N Am 20 (2009) 339–346
doi:10.1016/j.pmr.2008.12.004
1047-9651/08/$ – see front matter © 2009 Elsevier Inc. All rights reserved.

and from an upper middle-class background.[1,4] Additionally, a history of relatives suffering from chronic fatigue or a past medical history of asthma may be noted.[5] Emotional problems, such as anxiety or depression, can further increase the risk.[6] Associated symptoms can include headaches, muscle pains, fever, and exercise-induced fatigue.[7] Frequently, the illness is self-limited, but a minority of children may be persistently or severely affected.[8]

One reason for the failure of physicians to correctly diagnose this condition may be the child's inability to clearly articulate the chief complaint. Usually a parent concerned by the child's inactivity brings the matter to a physician's attention.[9] This clinical situation can be further compounded if the child suffers from a concurrent neuromuscular illness. Children with special health care needs may be most affected by chronic fatigue and least diagnosed. It is especially important to consider this disorder in such a specific population, as these children are often already delayed in physical and social function and, thus, stand to suffer worse outcomes.

DIFFERENTIATION OF FATIGUE VERSUS SLEEPINESS VERSUS WEAKNESS

Other symptoms such as sleepiness or weakness may be confused for chronic fatigue. It is important to differentiate fatigue from these separate entities as treatment may differ. This can prove difficult, because fatigue is a subjective and abstract concept. *Fatigue* implies an extreme mental and physical exhaustion independent of exertion, disease, or the amount of sleep,[10,11] whereas *sleepiness* implies a problem with the sleep/wake cycle itself.[11] Despite being separate entities, these 2 conditions can coexist.[11] *Weakness* more typically implies a defect in neuromuscular function.[9] This should be objectively measured by motor strength testing.

DIFFERENTIAL DIAGNOSIS

A vast array of diseases can imitate chronic fatigue (see **Table 1** for a noninclusive list of possible diagnoses). For this reason, it is imperative to rule out any active medical or psychiatric conditions that may lead to a misdiagnosis of chronic fatigue. It is advisable to perform a thorough history, including mental status examination, as well as a physical examination when evaluating a patient with fatigue. A minimum battery of laboratory screening tests, including complete blood count with leukocyte differential; erythrocyte sedimentation rate; electrolytes, alanine aminotransferase, total protein, albumin, alkaline phosphatase, calcium, phosphorus, glucose, blood urea nitrogen, and creatinine; thyroid-stimulating hormone; and urinalysis, should be performed.[10]

DEFINITION OF CHRONIC FATIGUE

Although chronic fatigue syndrome is an individual entity in the differential diagnosis of chronic fatigue, it may be helpful to examine this syndrome to formulate a working definition of chronic fatigue. According to the Centers for Disease Control and Prevention, to receive a diagnosis of chronic fatigue syndrome, a patient must satisfy 2 criteria:

1. Experience severe chronic fatigue for at least 6 months duration with no known causative medical conditions
2. Concurrently have at least 4 of the following symptoms: substantial impairment in short-term memory or concentration; sore throat; tender lymph nodes; muscle pain; multijoint pain without swelling or redness; headaches of a new type, pattern, or severity; lack of refreshing sleep; and postexertional malaise lasting more than 24 hours

Table 1 Differential diagnosis of chronic fatigue	
Cardiology arrhythmia	Chronic heart failure, cardiac defect
Endocrine	Cushing's disease, diabetes mellitus, obesity
ENT	Allergic rhinitis, sinusitis
GI Crohn's disease	Intussusception
ID	EBV, HIV, human herpes virus, lyme disease, parvovirus, polio
Neurology	Chronic fatigue syndrome, central fatigue, cerebral palsy, disseminated encephalomyelitis, multiple sclerosis, stroke, traumatic brain injury
Neuromuscular diseases	Amyotrophic lateral sclerosis, Charcot-Marie-Tooth disease, Guillan-Barré syndrome, immune neuropathy, myopathy, muscular dystrophy, myasthenia gravis, myotonic dystrophy
Oncology	Leukemia, lymphoma, solid tumor
Psychiatric	Anxiety, depression, psychosomatic disorders
Pulmonary	Cystic fibrosis, sarcoidosis, sleep-disordered breathing
Rheumatology	Fibromyalgia, juvenile rheumatoid arthritis, systemic lupus erythematosus

Abbreviations: EBV, Epstein-Barr virus; ENT, ear, nose, and throat; GI, gastrointestinal; HIV, human immunodeficiency virus; ID, infectious diseases.

These symptoms must be persistent or recurrent during the 6 or more consecutive months of illness. Additionally, they must not have predated the fatigue.[10]

Length of time is used to differentiate prolonged fatigue from chronic fatigue. Prolonged fatigue can be defined as lasting 1 month or longer, whereas chronic fatigue implies persistent or relapsing fatigue of 6 or more consecutive months.[10]

Although there is a significant research gap in the difference between chronic fatigue syndrome in children versus adults, there is 1 study that showed that outpatient rehabilitation significantly improved the prognosis of chronic fatigue syndrome in children and adolescents plagued with this illness.[12]

ANALYSIS OF FATIGUE SECONDARY TO NEUROLOGIC IMPAIRMENTS
Cerebral Palsy

Children with cerebral palsy (CP), especially the spastic variants, can be severely affected by fatigue. The mechanism behind fatigue in children with CP is not just on a muscular level but on a whole-body energy expenditure level. Fatigue consequently affects school function, home life, extracurricular activities, and socialization with peers.

Body mechanics as a whole in children with CP cause weakness to the affected muscles. However, on a single muscle level, limbs of children with CP actually show less fatigability. Studies comparing CP versus control muscles have shown that individual spastic muscles fatigue to a lesser extent than unaffected muscles.[13] It has been proposed that muscles affected with CP have an increase in type I muscle fibers. This is likely an adaptation to meet metabolic demands, as these muscles use the same motor units more repetitively and for longer durations during standing and ambulation.[13] Unfortunately, less fatigability on the single muscle level does not translate into less fatigue overall. On the contrary, spastic CP is associated with poorer functioning as well as with lower levels of activity and participation as measured by the gross motor function classification system.[14] Although agonist muscles are less fatigable individually, they also have a deficit in the volume of muscle activation, causing a decrease in force production.[13] Force is further affected by co-activation. When an agonist muscle fires, co-activation by the antagonist muscle has been observed. This also causes a decrease in peak force production.[13] Therefore, the combination of decreased muscle activation plus co-activation of antagonist muscles causes an overall weakness in children with CP.

The weakness of impaired biomechanical efficiency seen in CP also translates into a higher oxygen (O_2) requirement when comparing individuals with CP verses those without CP in matched activities.[14] For example, in a hemiplegic child versus a matched control, an activity such as walking will show a decrease in walking velocity, increased muscle weakness, decreased force production, and antagonist co-activation, all leading to higher O_2 requirements. Due to higher O_2 requirements, the child with CP will have an increase in energy expenditure and, therefore, be quicker to fatigue.[15]

Increase in muscle fatigue has not only been measured by energy expenditure but also by self-reporting from parents of children with CP. Studies have shown that children with a more severe diagnosis have an increased incidence of fatigue as reported by their parents.[16] Pain also appears to be a major contributor to fatigue with a direct correlation between the amount of pain and the amount of fatigue. There is also an inverse relationship between pain and fatigability and with quality of life (QOL) issues such as school functioning.[16]

Improvements in pain and prevention strategies of fatigability are ways to help improve the QOL in a child with CP. Treatment options for pain management and spasticity include muscle relaxants, such as botulinum toxin A, diazepam, and baclofen, as well as improvement of muscle strength and flexibility through physical therapy.[16] Fatigue-specific interventions often focus on decreasing energy expenditure. Adaptive equipment has been found to be particularly helpful in decreasing energy expenditure. Children with CP who require a wheelchair for mobility should be specially fitted with a customized wheelchair that takes the individual child's needs into consideration and subsequently provides them with the maximum upper-extremity function coupled with the most energy conservation.[16] If a child is ambulating but needs the assistance of a walker, studies have shown that although there is no difference in walking velocity or cadence between anterior and posterior walkers, there is an increase in upright positioning and decrease in oxygen consumption rates when a posterior walker is used.[17] Therefore, in terms of fatigability, a posterior walker would be recommended for energy conservation.[17] For the child ambulating without an assistive device, which is commonly seen in a child with hemiplegia, studies have shown that the addition of an ankle-foot-orthosis can be useful in controlling deformities, improving the child's gait efficiency from toe walking to a heel-toe gait, and subsequently reducing energy expenditure.[15] See **Table 2** for options in decreasing fatigue in children with CP.

Pediatric Multiple Sclerosis

According to the Multiple Sclerosis Council for Clinical Practice Guidelines,[18] Multiple sclerosis (MS)-related fatigue is defined as a "subjective lack of physical or mental energy that is perceived by the individual or caregiver to interfere with usual and desired activities" in patients with MS. Fatigue may be considered primary as opposed to secondary if it is unrelated to other MS symptoms. Primary fatigue, like other MS symptoms, may be worsened by heat and may precede a relapse.[18]

Patients most at risk for MS fatigue were generally older, affected by a more severe disability, and suffered from the progressive type of MS. Gender does not appear to

Table 2	
Options for reducing fatigue in children with cerebral palsy	
Pain Management	
Spasticity medications	Botulinum toxin A, diazepam, and baclofen
Adaptive equipment	Customized wheelchair, posterior walker
Orthosis	Ankle-foot-orthosis

have an association with the occurrence of fatigue in adults with MS. The occurrence of cerebellar signs had a positive correlation with fatigue; however, brain stem signs and visual and cognitive impairment did not.[19] Furthermore, fatigue severity does not appear to correlate with magnetic resonance imaging plaque load or atrophy assessed by conventional sequences.[20]

In children, MS is associated with cognitive impairment and low IQ scores in addition to fatigue. A younger age at onset correlated with the severity of low IQ.[21]

Treatment with modafinil has been shown to significantly improve fatigue and sleepiness in patients with MS. It is generally well tolerated and is effective at a lower dose in MS patients than that used in the regimen for patients with narcolepsy.[22] There has also been support for the fact that amantadine, an antiviral agent, is significantly better than placebo in treating fatigue in MS patients.[23]

One study demonstrated that an extended outpatient rehabilitation program for patients with progressive MS effectively reduced fatigue and the severity of other symptoms. No statistically significant impact on functional status was shown; however, there appeared to be less loss function in the treatment group compared with that in the control group.[24]

Heat is known to increase the frequency and severity of clinical signs and symptoms of MS. One study has shown that precooling the patients in cool water was effective in preventing an increase in core body temperature with physical work. This method may enable heat-sensitive individuals with MS to exercise with greater physical comfort.[25]

Post-Polio Syndrome

Children with neuromuscular illness can continue to experience complications including chronic fatigue as adults. One such illness, polio, often manifests itself in childhood but does not lead to fatigue until in adulthood. Post-polio syndrome (PPS) refers to the new development of neuromuscular symptoms, including muscle weakness and fatigue in skeletal or bulbar muscles, unrelated to any known cause, that begins many years after an acute attack of paralytic poliomyelitis.[26]

Criteria defined by Post-Polio Health International to identify PPS include (1) a confirmed history of polio, (2) neurologic and functional recovery after the acute episode followed by at least 15 years of neurologic and functional stability, (3) the gradual onset of extensive fatigue, muscle and/or joint pain, new weakness in muscles, and/or new muscle atrophy, and (4) the exclusion of any other medical explanation.[27]

Although the cause of PPS remains controversial, there is some support that the new signs and symptoms are due in part to an excessive metabolic stress on the remaining motor neurons. This results in premature degeneration of surviving motor neurons with the loss of axonal terminals.[28]

One hypothesis for treating fatigue in PPS is to use medication that alleviates daytime somnolence. However, studies of the use of modafinil did not show effectiveness in alleviating the symptoms of fatigue in PPS patients.[29]

Treatment of PPS includes select exercise programs, gait aids (walking sticks, crutches, wheelchairs), orthotics (ankle-foot orthosis), adaptive equipment (long-handled aids and grabbers, rails in bathroom), and lifestyle changes (rest breaks, part-time work) with focused treatment of specific symptoms, such as fatigue, weakness, pain, and bulbar dysfunction.[30]

Psychiatric Illness

Psychological factors may contribute to the cause and persistence of adolescent chronic fatigue. One study showed that adolescents with profound chronic fatigue reported more somatic symptoms and missed more school days as a result of their symptoms than those of adolescents referred for migraine. Additionally, fatigued adolescents showed higher depressive symptom scores than those of adolescents without fatigue.[31]

Pediatric-Onset Spinal Cord Injury

Individuals with SCI are typically young at the time of injury and experience an immediate reduction in their functional reserves and capacities. Young children require extra time to achieve upper body strength to propel a wheelchair for maximum independence in various settings. The skeletally immature child with weakness and spasticity may develop orthopedic problems during growth, such as hip subluxation and scoliosis which may result in altered function and fatigue with sitting and ambulation. As growth in stature further increases high energy demands of walking, many children who were partial ambulators choose to give up walking for fulltime wheelchair use around adolescence. Obesity, attributed to reduced energy expenditure related to muscle paralysis, decreased lean body mass and lower physical activity levels, may lead to early fatigue and further restriction of activities.[32]

Several investigations have identified symptom patterns that herald the onset of a functional impairment syndrome in persons with SCI, similar to what is described in polio survivors. Nonactivity-dependent fatigue is reported by 61%, followed by new pain and weakness in 31–36%. Individuals injured during or before adolescence enjoy a maintenance phase of 20 years before experiencing functional decline. Losses in function result in difficulty performing skills previously mastered, increased need for personal assistance, equipment and rehabilitation services.[33]

Activity modifications to preserve upper extremity function at an early age may include weight bearing with a neutral wrist position instead of extended wrist, and performing side-to-side or forward lean pressure reliefs instead of wheelchair pushups. The use of splinting and adaptive equipment such as overhead reachers and sliding boards can minimize shoulder impingement positions. Adapting the wheelchair with flex rims and using gel-padded gloves may provide shock absorption from repetitive wheel contact and a better grip on the pushrim. Suboptimal posture-related fatigue may be amenable to wheelchair seating system modifications. Maintenance of equipment is another important factor because low tire pressure and misaligned wheels contribute to increased rolling resistance. Instruction in energy conservation techniques, pacing with rest periods and use of pushrim-activated power assist wheels can reduce the physiologic demand of manual wheelchair propulsion.[33]

Needs for new equipment may not be well recognized by the parents or primary healthcare providers of children with SCI. Multidisciplinary collaboration within a medical home model that incorporates continuity of care, collaboration with specialists, regularly scheduled communication with school/home therapists as well as community service coordinators, can facilitate timely identification of changing functional needs and the resources to acquire appropriate equipment to prevent secondary complications.

SUMMARY

Children with neuromuscular illness are at high risk for fatigue. This symptom, although difficult to decipher, can contribute significantly to the child's disability. It is, therefore, imperative to consider fatigue in the management of children with special health care needs. Currently, the literature on chronic fatigue in children is sparse and so more investigative work must be done to understand and manage this condition.

REFERENCES

1. Carter BD, Edwards JF, Kronenberger WG, et al. Case control study of chronic fatigue in pediatric patients. Pediatrics 1995;95(2):179–86.
2. Garralda ME, Rangel L. Annotation: chronic fatigue syndrome in children and adolescents. J Child Psychol Psychiatry 2002;43:169–76. Doi:10.1111/1469-7610.00010.
3. Farmer A, Fowler T, Scourfield J, et al. Prevalence of chronic disabling fatigue in children and adolescents. Br J Psychiatry 2004;184:477–81. Doi:10.1192/bjp.184.6.477.
4. Carter BD, Marshall GS. New developments: diagnosis and management of chronic fatigue in children and adolescents. Curr Probl Pediatr 1995;25:281–93.
5. Bell KM, Cookfair D, Bell DS, et al. Risk factors associated with chronic fatigue syndrome in a cluster of pediatric cases. Rev Infect Dis 1991;13(Suppl 1):S32–8.
6. Rimes KA, Goodman R, Hotopf M, et al. Incidence, prognosis, and risk factors for fatigue and chronic fatigue syndrome in adolescents: a prospective community study. Pediatrics 2007;119(3):e603–9.
7. Mears CJ, Taylor RR, Jordan KM, et al. Pediatric Practice Research Group. Socio-demographic and symptom correlates of fatigue in an adolescent primary care sample. J Adolesc Health 2004;35(6):528e 21–6.
8. Marshall GS, Gesser RM, Yamanishi K, et al. Chronic fatigue in children: clinical features, Epstein-Barr virus and human herpes virus 6 serology and long term follow-up. Pediatr Infect Dis J 1991;10:287–90.
9. Hoekelman RA, Mosby I. Primary pediatric care. 4th edition. St. Louis (MO): Mosby; 2001.
10. Fukuda K, Straus SE, Hickie I, et al. The chronic fatigue syndrome: a comprehensive approach to its definition and study. International Chronic Fatigue Syndrome Study Group. Ann Intern Med 1994;121:953–9.
11. Shen J, Barbera J, Shapiro CM. Distinguishing sleepiness and fatigue: focus on definition and measurement. Sleep Med Rev 2006;10(1):63–76.
12. Viner R, Gregorowski A, Wine C, et al. Outpatient rehabilitative treatment of chronic fatigue syndrome (CFS/ME). Arch Dis Child 2004;89(7):615–9.
13. Stackhouse S, Binder-Macleod S, Lee S. Voluntary muscle activation, contractile properties, and fatigability in children with and without cerebral palsy. Muscle Nerve 2005;31:594–601.
14. Moreau N, Li L, Geaghan J, et al. Fatigue resistance during a voluntary performance task is associated with lower levels of mobility in cerebral palsy. Arch Phys Med Rehabil 2008;89(10):2011–6.
15. Balaban B, Yasar E, Dal U, et al. The effect of hinged ankle-foot orthosis on gait and energy expenditure in spastic hemiplegic cerebral palsy. Disabil Rehabil 2007;29(2):139–44.

16. Berrin S, Malcarne V, Varni J, et al. Pain, fatigue, and school functioning in children with cerebral palsy: a path-analytic model. J Pediatr Psychol 2007;32(3): 330–7.
17. Stavness C. The effect of positioning for children with cerebral palsy on upper-extremity function: a review of the evidence. Phys Occup Ther Pediatr 2006; 26(3):39–53.
18. Multiple Sclerosis Council for Clinical Practice Guidelines. Fatigue and multiple sclerosis: evidence-based management strategies for fatigue in multiple sclerosis. Washington, DC: Paralyzed Veterans of America; 1998.
19. Colosimo C, Millefiorini E, Grasso MG, et al. Fatigue in MS is associated with specific clinical features. Acta Neurol Scand 1995;92(5):353–5.
20. Bakshi R, Miletich RS, Henschel K, et al. Fatigue in multiple sclerosis: cross-sectional correlation with brain MRI findings in 71 patients. Neurology 1999; 53(5):1151–3.
21. Amato MP, Goretti B, Ghezzi A, et al. Cognitive and psychosocial features of childhood and juvenile MS. Neurology 2008;70(20):1891–7.
22. Zifko UA, Rupp M, Schwarz S, et al. Modafinil in treatment of fatigue in multiple sclerosis. Results of an open-label study. J Neurol 2002;249(8):983–7.
23. Krupp LB, Coyle PK, Doscher C, et al. Fatigue therapy in multiple sclerosis: results of a double-blind, randomized, parallel trial of amantadine, pemoline, and placebo. Neurology 1995;45(11):1956–61.
24. Di Fabio RP, Soderberg J, Choi T, et al. Extended outpatient rehabilitation: its influence on symptom frequency, fatigue, and functional status for persons with progressive multiple sclerosis. Arch Phys Med Rehabil 1998;79(2):141–6.
25. White AT, Wilson TE, Davis SL, et al. Effect of precooling on physical performance in multiple sclerosis. Mult Scler 2000;6(3):176–80.
26. Dalakas MC. The post-polio syndrome as an evolved clinical entity. Definition and clinical description. Ann N Y Acad Sci 1995;753:68–80.
27. Laurie G, Maynard FM, Fischer DA, et al. Handbook on the Late Effects of Polio-myelitis for Physicians and Survivors. 1st edition. Gazette International Networking Institute; 1984. p. 5.
28. Grimby G, Stalberg E, Sandberg A, et al. An 8-year longitudinal study of muscle strength, muscle fiber size, and dynamic electromyogram in individuals with late polio. Muscle Nerve 1998;21:1428–37.
29. Chan KM, Strohschein FJ, Rydz D, et al. Randomized controlled trial of modafinil for the treatment of fatigue in postpolio patients. Muscle Nerve 2006;33(1): 138–41.
30. Khan F. Rehabilitation for postpolio sequelae. Aust Fam Physician 2004;33(8): 621–4.
31. Smith MS, Martin-Herz SP, Womack WM, et al. Comparative study of anxiety, depression, somatization, functional disability, and illness attribution in adolescents with chronic fatigue or migraine. Pediatrics 2003;111(4 Pt 1):e376–81.
32. Molnar G, Murphy K. Spina Bifida. In: Molnar G, Alexander M, editors. Pediatric Rehabilitation. Hanley and Belfus; 1998. p. 219–45.
33. Capoor J, Stein AB. Aging with spinal cord injury. Phys Med Rehabil Clin N Am 2005;16:129–61.

Fatigue in Parkinson Disease, Stroke, and Traumatic Brain Injury

Jaime Levine, DO[a],*, Brian D. Greenwald, MD[b]

KEYWORDS

- Fatigue • Traumatic brain injury • Parkinson disease • Stroke
- Cerebrovascular accident • Post-stroke syndrome

Fatigue is a commonly reported symptom after traumatic brain injury (TBI), after stroke, and in persons living with Parkinson disease (PD). Fatigue compounds the underlying impairments of all these neurologic disabilities, leading to greater handicap and lower life satisfaction. Fatigue in neurologic illnesses has serious social and public health implications. One study looking at social security disability insurance (SSDI) in PD found that 82% of patients in their sample felt they were too disabled to work full-time at a mean of 3.4 years after PD diagnosis.[1] The primary debilitating symptom that contributed to applying for SSDI in this study was fatigue.

Merriam-Webster's Collegiate Dictionary defines fatigue as "weariness or exhaustion from labor, exertion or stress; the temporary loss of power to respond that is induced in a sensory receptor or motor end organ by continued stimulation," and tiredness is defined as, "the state of being drained of strength and energy; fatigued often to the point of exhaustion." In laypersons' terms, they are synonyms. Medical literature generally employs yet another similar definition, describing fatigue as a *subjectively* overwhelming sense of tiredness, lack of energy, and feeling of exhaustion. These similar definitions are all irrespective of sleep status.

It is important to note that people with neurologic disorders describe fatigue differently from the way that the general population does. One paramount distinction is that fatigue experienced by individuals with neurologic disorders does not respond to sleep or rest nor is it accompanied by the *desire* to sleep, whereas people in the general population report an amelioration of fatigue symptoms with a nap or a full night's sleep. This important difference in definitions has implications for research, because scales used to quantify fatigue in the general population may not accurately measure fatigue in those with neurologic conditions.

---

[a] Department of Physical Medicine and Rehabilitation, St. Vincent's Medical Center, 170 West 12th Street, Link 103, New York, NY 10011, USA
[b] Mount Sinai Medical Center, Department of Rehabilitation Medicine, 5 East 98th Street, Box 1240B, New York, NY 10029, USA
* Corresponding author.
E-mail address: rehabdoc@mac.com (J. Levine).

Phys Med Rehabil Clin N Am 20 (2009) 347–361
doi:10.1016/j.pmr.2008.12.006
1047-9651/08/$ – see front matter © 2009 Elsevier Inc. All rights reserved.

Although there is no universally accepted definition for fatigue, there is a general distinction between peripheral and central fatigue. Peripheral fatigue, or physical fatigue, is most commonly expressed as musculoskeletal symptoms that impair mobility and the ability to perform activities of daily living (ADLs).

Central fatigue, also known as mental or cognitive fatigue, results from dysfunction of the supratentorial structure involved in performing cognitive tasks. Central fatigue is a difficulty initiating and sustaining mental and physical tasks in the absence of motor or physical impairments.[2,3] The inability to maintain focused attention is a key component of central fatigue, since focused attention is necessary to incorporate the mental, physical, and sensory inputs involved in completing a task. Once focused attention is impaired, integrating the various types of information needed to complete a task becomes more difficult and requires greater effort to complete.

In persons with TBI and stroke, central fatigue predominates, whereas in PD, fatigue complaints are often mixed. In evaluating patients with complaints of fatigue, differentiating between central and peripheral fatigue is an important initial step, as inciting agents and treatments differ between the 2. The goal of this article is to provide the reader with an overview of the etiology, assessment, quality of life (QoL) implications, and treatment of this common symptom in adults with neurologic disabilities.

EPIDEMIOLOGY

Fatigue is reported to be almost ubiquitous in individuals with neurologic disorders. Estimates of prevalence depend somewhat on the specific neurologic disorder in question, the scale used, and the study cited. Additionally, as discussed, the definition of fatigue tends to vary from study to study, so statistics cannot always be directly compared. Regardless, it is accepted that fatigue is an extremely common problem associated with neurologic disorders, which is reported with significantly higher frequency than that in the general population and may significantly affect an individual's return to independent living.

Fatigue can be a debilitating symptom of PD, affecting all aspects of life. Although the literature studying fatigue in PD lags behind that of other neurologic entities, it has recently begun to flourish. The prevalence of fatigue in PD varies in the literature from 33% to 81%. Two important studies done in 1993 were among the first to highlight the relationship between fatigue and PD.[4,5] These studies reported for the first time that the rate of fatigue in PD was high. In the study by Friedman and colleagues, more than 50% of their PD patients reported that fatigue was among the 3 most disabling symptoms of their disease. This is important to keep in mind, because physicians on the whole are not doing an adequate job of recognizing fatigue in their PD patients. In 1 study, 42% of patients with PD complained of fatigue, whereas only 25% of the physicians uncovered the symptom.[6]

Fatigue as an *independent* symptom in PD is a relatively new concept. Karlsen and colleagues[7] were the first to present evidence backing the claim that the high prevalence of fatigue seen in PD cannot be explained by comorbid depression, dementia, or sleep disorders alone. Alves and colleagues[8] studied PD patients for 8 years, measuring the prevalence of fatigue at the inception of the study and 4 and 8 years later. They found that the prevalence of fatigue in patients without depression and excessive daytime sleepiness remained high and increased from 32.1% to 38.9% during the 8-year study period.

The prevalence of fatigue after stroke ranges from 30% to 68%.[9] Fatigue is reported both in the acute phase and the late phase after stroke. Ingles and colleagues[10] found that fatigue problems, measured by the Fatigue Impact Scale (FIS), were reported in

68% of subjects between 3 and 13 months after stroke, compared to 36% of age-matched control subjects. Two years after stroke, 51% of survivors have elevated scores on the fatigue subscale of the Checklist Individual Strength compared to 12% of control subjects, and 50% report that fatigue is their main complaint. Controlling for depression, 39.2% of stroke survivors experience significant fatigue independent of reports of depression. In addition, the frequency of fatigue associated with clinically relevant depression was found to be 67% in individuals who had strokes at least 7 years earlier.

A 2006 study tracked the natural history of post-stroke fatigue for 1 year.[11] The authors used the Fatigue Severity Scale (FSS) to measure fatigue at admission, 6 months, and then 1 year after stroke. They found that the incidence of fatigue increased with each subsequent evaluation and that fatigue impact was greater among women, older subjects, and those who exhibited more depressive symptoms.

There is no clear primary etiology of fatigue after TBI. Depression, pain, sleep disturbance, and neuroendocrine abnormalities all have been associated with fatigue after TBI.[12–14] It has also been hypothesized that the injured brain requires more effort to compensate for impairments in attention and processing speed.[15–17] Many individuals with TBI describe mental tasks as being effortful and fatiguing.

Fatigue is a commonly experienced symptom after TBI and occurs at a greater frequency than that in the general population.[15] Fatigue is among the most pervasive symptoms after TBI.[18,19] Estimates of the incidence of fatigue in individuals living in the community range from 50% to 80%.[20] Fatigue after TBI appears to be independent of severity and age at time of injury and is associated with duration after TBI in some studies and not others.[15,21] In a 2-year prospective longitudinal study by Bushnik and colleagues[22] of individuals with moderate to severe TBI, improvements in fatigue were seen in the first year. Further changes were not seen up to 2 years after TBI. The subset of individuals who reported significant increases in fatigue during the first 2 years demonstrated poorer outcomes in multiple domains than did those with stable or decreased fatigue.

EFFECTS ON QUALITY OF LIFE
Parkinson Disease

Patients with PD have worse QoL scores compared with those of the general population, and PD patients with fatigue have even lower scores. A shifting focus from defining the symptoms of this disease to describing their QoL implications is reflected in current literature. It is well known that fatigue is rated among the most disabling symptoms of PD, but it was not until recently that we knew how this symptom compared with other common symptoms. A 2008 British study looked at the *relative* importance of symptoms with respect to QoL in PD patients and found that fatigue was as important as some of the classic motor symptoms, such as shuffling and falls.[23]

A well-done Slovakian study used several scales to measure the effects that fatigue has on QoL in PD patients.[24] The authors found that the existence of fatigue in PD patients was associated with lower scores on all QoL domains, the most affected being bodily discomfort, mobility, and emotional well-being. In addition, a 2003 Norwegian study described the influence of fatigue on health-related QoL in patients with PD.[25] The authors' sample included patients without known depression or dementia, and they used the FSS as a measuring tool. They found that 50% of the patients had significant fatigue and that those with fatigue had a more advanced disease than those without. They also uncovered a strong correlation between fatigue and high distress scores on health-related QoL scales.

Stroke

Fatigue in a post-stroke patient can have significant QoL-lowering effects. Van de Port and colleagues[26] were the first to show that fatigue is an independent variable in post-stroke patients. They also found that post-stroke fatigue is more closely related to instrumental activities of daily living (IADLs), such as shopping and cleaning, than to simple ADLs. Another study found that health-related QoL in patients who survived an ischemic stroke was lowest in the domain of physical mobility.[27] It is not surprising that fatigue is predictive of mobility decline 1 year after stroke,[28] yet the relationship between ambulatory activity and post-stroke fatigue is complex. Several other studies have shown no relationship between mobility and fatigue or daily step activity and fatigue,[29,30] yet it is clear to all that the 2 have a relationship. It is likely that more salient variables such as hemiparesis or social isolation become the primary obstacles to mobility after stroke.

Traumatic Brain Injury

Cantor and colleagues studied community dwelling individuals who had suffered a range of severity of TBI to examine the relationships between post-TBI fatigue and comorbid conditions, participation in activities, QoL, and demographic and injury variables. A noninjured control group was also examined. Fatigue was more severe and prevalent in individuals with TBI and more severe among women. It was not correlated with other demographic and injury variables. Fatigue was correlated with health-related QoL and overall QoL but was not generally related to participation in major life activities.[31]

DIFFERENTIAL DIAGNOSIS

Fatigue should always be suspected and inquired about when encountering a patient with a neurologic condition, yet it is critical to keep in mind that the patient's fatigue may not be due to that neurologic condition. It is important to determine whether the fatigue is primary or in fact secondary to another condition. The differential diagnosis for fatigue is vast, but **Table 1** provides a summary of the most common non-neurologic causes of fatigue.

The issues of fatigue and disordered sleep are closely intertwined, and differentiating the 2 is often a problem for physicians. Although sleep disorders are common in many neurologic conditions, it is believed that fatigue itself is an independent symptom, often unexplained by a comorbid sleep disorder. Though they share common symptomatology, the treatments are quite different. It is a challenge to the physician to disentangle this perplexing constellation of symptoms and determine the root of the problem so that proper therapy can then be administered. Depression is another entity common in both the general population and among those with neurologic diseases. As with sleep disorders, it is possible that a patient's fatigue is not primary but secondary to comorbid depression. Another important thing to remember is that dementia occurs in 10% to 15% of PD patients, so it is important not to neglect this possibility in your differential diagnosis of fatigue.[32]

ASSESSMENT

When evaluating any patient with symptoms of fatigue, it is crucial to conduct a thorough diagnostic workup looking for underlying causes that may be unrelated to any known neurologic diagnoses. Initially, the clinician should attempt to differentiate between central and peripheral origins as well as primary versus secondary causes.

Table 1
Differential diagnosis of fatigue
Neuropsychiatric
Depression
Sleep disorders
Dementia
Infectious
Endocrine
Hypothyroidism
Anterior pituitary dysfunction
Hypogonadism
Growth hormone deficiency
Adrenal insufficiency
Chronic disease
Diabetes
Cardiac disease
Pulmonary disease
Anemia
Cancer
Hepatorenal disease
Rheumatologic disease
Medications
Antispasticity agents & muscle relaxants
Analgesics
Anticonvulsants
Antihistamines
Anti-inflammatories
Antipsychotics
Antidepressants
Gastrointestinal drugs

Central fatigue questioning and examination typically focus on the presence of fatigue when attempting to perform cognitive tasks that require 1 or more steps. Peripheral fatigue questions focus on fatigue with physical activities such as walking, lifting, or completing ADLs.

It is also important to think in terms of primary and secondary causes for fatigue. Primary fatigue is caused by the neurologic disorder itself, whereas secondary fatigue can be due to multiple factors such as anemia, lack of conditioning, depression, side effects of medications, infection, endocrine dysfunction, or sleep disturbance (**Table 2**). Many medications can cause fatigue as a side effect, and examples are listed in **Table 1**. Checking serum levels of some medications and review of medications for interactions should be a part of the compulsory evaluation of fatigue. In assessing for secondary causes of fatigue, inquiring about current medications, difficulties sleeping, and depression can also yield useful information.

Evaluation for sleep disturbance is a core component in evaluating the etiology of the fatigue. High rates of sleep disturbance have been shown to be associated with

Table 2
Patient assessment of fatigue

Ascertain type of fatigue
- Mental fatigue: Fatigue with cognitive tasks
- Physical fatigue: Fatigue with walking, lifting, and other activities of daily living

Evaluate for secondary causes of fatigue (See Table 1)
- Assess for depression
- Sleep dysfunction
  - Sleep onset
  - Staying asleep
  - Nightmares
- Infection
  - Fever
  - Chills
  - Sweats
  - Urinary symptoms
- Underlying malignancy
  - Weight loss
  - Loss of appetite
  - Anemia

Careful review of medications
- Side effects
- Drug–drug interactions

Laboratory and imaging studies when appropriate

all neurologic disabilities, although for varying reasons. Management of sleep impairment through sleep hygiene, treatment of comorbid illness, or through pharmacology can decrease fatigue. Depression is often associated with disturbances in sleep, appetite, concentration, as well as fatigue.

Hematologic, infectious, endocrine, cardiac, rheumatologic, and metabolic causes of fatigue should be considered. History and physical will help guide the workup, but laboratory testing for metabolic and endocrine function should be standard.

Anterior pituitary dysfunction has been documented after TBI, stroke, and diagnosis of PD. Endocrine dysfunction has been shown to be as high as 59% after TBI.[33] Growth hormone deficiency and hypogonadism are associated with decreased bone mineral densities, aerobic capacity, muscle strength, lower QoL, cognitive impairments, as well as fatigue.[34] Basic screening for endocrine dysfunction should include a thyroid panel, AM cortisol, testosterone, facioscapulohumeral dystrophy, and luteinizing hormone as appropriate, and insulin-like growth factor-1 as a marker of growth hormone. The relationship between fatigue and neuroendocrine dysfunction is still evolving.

A driving assessment should be a routine part of any patient encounter when fatigue is an issue. Driving safety is a controversial issue without clear guidelines in this population, and specific recommendations are often left to the careful discretion of physicians. There is a small but important body of literature looking at the effects that fatigue in PD has on driving. One study assessed the effects of auditory-verbal distraction on driving performance in PD, showing that drivers with PD made more errors during baseline and with distraction than did their counterparts without the disease.[35] In this study, daytime sleepiness predicted worsening of driving due to distraction. Another study questioned PD patients about occurrences of sudden onset of sleep at the wheel (SOS).[36] Their alarming results showed that of the patients holding a driver's license, 15% had experienced SOS at the wheel in the past 5 years, and in 11% of cases, the episode led to an accident. The risk of accidents in this study was correlated with an increased score on the Epworth Sleepiness Scale (ESS).

Parkinson Disease

When evaluating already-diagnosed PD patients, it is important not to allow their motor symptoms, including bradykinesia, resting tremor, rigidity, and postural insta- bility, to monopolize an office visit. Studies have shown that nonmotor symptoms of PD, such as fatigue, can have just as negative an impact on QoL as motor symp- toms.[37] It is also important to keep in mind that there is no clear correlation between the severity of motor symptoms and the presence or severity of fatigue, so the clinician must ask about nonmotor symptoms even in PD patients without severe motor symp- toms. There is evidence that the presence of nonmotor symptoms may actually predict the development of PD. In fact, fatigue is usually encountered early in the disease, often before an official diagnosis of PD is made.[38]

It is well known that patients with PD already walk at a slower speed, have increased episodes of fall, and have less of an ability to multitask while walking than those without the disease. Contributing to this body of knowledge, 1 study showed that performance of additional tasks while walking resulted in a reduction of walking speed and mean step length in PD patients over the general population.[39] Physical fatigue showed a significant relationship with gait speed in this study; however, it was balance that accounted for most of the variance in walking speed. Another study found that increased levels of fatigue were associated with decreased levels of leisure physical activity, lower frequency of vigorous physical activity, and less time performing ADLss.[40] This relationship between activity and fatigue in PD patients remains unclear, however. One study showed that although PD patients experience significantly greater levels of fatigue than those of controls for a given amount of physical activity, this was not associated with a decrease in physical activity when given the opportunity.[41] These data underscore the fact that an assessment of physical activity level and exer- cise tolerance should be part of every fatigue evaluation.

Stroke

Assessment of fatigue in post-stroke patients is perhaps the most difficult of all neuro- logic entities because many patients will have trouble distinguishing peripheral fatigue from muscle weakness secondary to the stroke. Careful use of language and good communication are especially important while conducting this interview.

Lynch and colleagues[42] propose case definitions of post-stroke fatigue, which correlated well with substantially higher fatigue scores on 4 common FSSs. They differentiated between patients in the community and hospitalized patients. Their proposed case definition for post-stroke fatigue in community patients is "Over the past month, there has been at least a 2-week period when patient has experienced fatigue, a lack of energy, or an increased need to rest every day or nearly every day. This fatigue has led to difficulty taking part in everyday activities."

It is important not to neglect the possibility of post-stroke fatigue in patients who have had mild strokes. Carlsson and colleagues[43] showed that after mild stroke involving minimal or no motor or cognitive impairments, 75% of their subjects still stated that their stroke affected everyday life. Astheno-emotional disorder (AED), with fatigue being the most important symptom, was found in 72% of the sample. Carlsson and colleagues[44] went on to further characterize AED the following year and concluded that although fatigue was a pervasive element of this syndrome, it was often hidden to others. This finding highlights the importance of asking about this symptom during office visits.

Traumatic Brain Injury

In the assessment of fatigue after TBI, high yield correlates that require evaluation and treatment include sleep disturbance, hormonal disorders, and pain.

Insomnia, or difficulty initiating or maintaining sleep, is reported with a frequency of 27% to 70% or higher in those with higher frequencies early post injury.[45,46] Disordered sleep can have adverse behavioral, physical, and cognitive consequences. Endocrine dysfunction has been shown to be as high as 59% after TBI.[33] Growth hormone deficiency and hypogonadism are associated with decreased bone mineral densities, aerobic capacity, muscle strength, lower QoL, and cognitive impairments as well as fatigue.[34] The relationship between fatigue and neuroendocrine dysfunction is still evolving.

Scales

Several scales are available to help quantify the magnitude and impact of fatigue in general. Some of the more commonly used scales include the FSS (see **Table 3**), the ESS, the FIS, and the Modified Fatigue Impact Scale (MFIS). In the FSS, the patient is asked to rate 9 statements about fatigue on the degree of agreement, and then the score is averaged. People with depression alone score about 4.5, but people with fatigue related to multiple sclerosis (MS), for example, average about 6.5. The ESS measures the likelihood of a subject dozing during certain mundane daily activities, such as watching television or being a passenger in a car ride lasting for 1 hour. The test subjects must rate each activity based on how likely they feel they would be able to doze off while engaged in that activity. The FIS is a 40-item questionnaire that separates functional categories into physical, cognitive, and psychosocial subsets. Each question is rated 1 to 4. The MFIS is a shorter, 21-item derivative of the FIS and has most frequently been used in the MS population.

One possible reason for the slow pace of research on fatigue in PD is the lack of simple tools available to measure fatigue in this population. The Parkinson Fatigue

Table 3
Fatigue severity scale
Each statement is rated 1 to 7. 1 indicates strong disagreement, and 7 indicates strong agreement
1. My motivation is lower when I am fatigued.
2. Exercise brings on my fatigue.
3. I am easily fatigued.
4. Fatigue interferes with my physical functioning.
5. Fatigue causes frequent problems for me.
6. My fatigue prevents sustained physical functioning.
7. Fatigue interferes with carrying out certain duties and responsibilities.
8. Fatigue is among my 3 most disabling symptoms.
9. Fatigue interferes with my work, family, or social life.

Scale (PFS) attempts to fill that niche by providing a quick and reliable tool physicians can use to assess fatigue, specifically in PD patients. The PFS is a 16-item questionnaire arising from statements made by PD patients with fatigue, such as, "I get tired more quickly than other people I know," and "Everything I do is an effort." Although the full scope of this scale's utility is yet to be determined, the PFS will certainly facilitate future research on this topic.

There are 4 scales that are commonly used to measure post-stroke fatigue: The Fatigue Assessment Scale (FAS), the general subscale of the Multidimensional Fatigue Symptom Inventory, the fatigue subscale of the Profile of Mood States, and the Brief Fatigue Inventory. A recent comparison of these fatigue scales determined that although all 4 were valid and feasible to use in stroke patients, the FAS was most highly recommended, because it had the best test-retest reliability.[47] The FAS is a 10-item, self-administered questionnaire consisting of statements describing aspects of fatigue, which the subject must rate according to their agreement. Examples include "Physically, I am exhausted," and "I have problems thinking clearly."

The Newcastle Stroke-Specific Quality of Life Measure (NEWSQOL) was recently developed to specifically measure QoL in stroke patients across 11 domains.[48] Among these domains are sleep, cognition, and fatigue. The NEWSQOL is an interviewer-administered multiple-choice questionnaire, with questions varying according to domain. Examples of the fatigue questions include "Do you doze off during the day because of the stroke?" and "Because of the stroke, are there days when you feel you could sleep all the time?" The subjects are then asked to respond with, "no, occasionally, sometimes, or always." This scale has shown evidence of reliability and validity and is a promising tool for quantifying QoL after stroke.

The Global Fatigue Index is a widely used measure of fatigue in multiple populations including TBI.[31] It is derived from 15 of 16 items of the Multidimensional Assessment of Fatigue (MAF).[49] The MAF covers 4 domains: severity, distress, impact on ADLs, and timing.

TREATMENT

The treatment of fatigue can be broadly divided into pharmacologic and nonpharmacologic interventions. Pharmacologic interventions include medications, hormone replacement, and herbal remedies. These are discussed below. Nonpharmacologic treatments include patient and caregiver education, psychological approaches, osteopathic manipulative therapy, and physical exercise.

Pharmacologic Interventions

Several classes of medications have been demonstrated to be effective for the treatment of fatigue after neurologic disease or injury. Primarily among these are the classic neurostimulants, other wakefulness-promoting agents, and antidepressants. Many anecdotal reports exist for other medications for fatigue. However, as with most issues regarding the pharmacologic treatment of symptoms following neurologic disorders, there is scant objective research studying the effects these medications have on fatigue. The information below is not intended to be a comprehensive list but rather to offer some broad information about typical prescribing practices for this problem.

Classic neurostimulants are probably the most widely studied medications for fatigue following a multitude of disorders, including cancer, PD, TBI, and stroke. In a comparison study with sertraline, methylphenidate was found to be more efficacious for daytime sleepiness on the ESS in patients with TBI.[50] Another recent study showed that methylphenidate improves fatigue scores on the FSS in PD following a 6-week treatment period.[51] An additional benefit of methylphenidate in the PD population is its ability to potentiate the effects of L-dopa, thus increasing the "on" time.[52] Other neurostimulants that have been used clinically include dextroamphetamine, pemoline, and mixed amphetamine-dextroamphetamine salts. Most of these medications have broad effects of increasing the activity of, or stimulating receptors of, endogenous adrenergic or cholinergic receptors. This has a general effect on patient's subjective feeling of wakefulness and may also have other cognitive effects, such as improving attention and concentration.

Modafinil has been widely used as an agent to combat fatigue. Modafinil is indicated for the treatment of narcolepsy and daytime somnolence. Although anecdotal reports suggest that it is helpful in treating fatigue in TBI, a controlled study by Jha and colleagues[53] failed to show consistent patterns of relief of fatigue in a brain-injured population. Modafinil has also been studied in PD, although in a recent study it failed to significantly improve excessive daytime sleepiness in this population.[54] Despite this lack of scientific evidence, it remains a widely used drug for treatment of fatigue in stroke, TBI, and PD.

Dopaminergic medications, especially amantadine, have been used as medications for arousal following TBI, PD, MS, and stroke. Amantadine has garnered significant research attention in the MS population and has been shown to be clinically effective in combating fatigue when compared with placebo.[55] Dopamine agonists are also becoming increasingly more important in the treatment of PD, though there is no clear evidence of their effect on fatigue. In fact a recent study found that fatigue in PD was not influenced by dopamine agonists.[56] Case reports have found amantadine to be useful in mutism, apathy, inattention, and impulsivity after TBI. Amantadine appears to have positive effects on arousal, agitation, and cognition after TBI but studies of its use in fatigue after TBI are lacking.[57]

Levodopa is likely the most effective medication in controlling the motor symptoms in PD, yet its effects on fatigue are not well studied. There is 1 study, however, that indirectly demonstrates that levodopa is actually effective in reducing physical fatigue as measured by finger tapping, a commonly used measure of PD severity.[58]

Traditional antidepressant medications, especially selective serotonin reuptake inhibitors, have also been medications of interest. Paroxetine has been reported as an agent to combat fatigue following TBI, MS, and stroke; however, its use has not been strongly identified for the treatment of fatigue in the absence of depressive symptoms. In addition, in that class, a recent double-blind, placebo-controlled study done in South Korea showed that although decreasing post-stroke depression, Fluoxetine was not effective in lessening post-stroke fatigue.[59]

The tricyclic antidepressants, mainly amitriptyline, have also been reported to be effective for fatigue, although the effects noted are more likely a result of improved sleep patterns and decreased vegetative symptoms of depression, rather than the true dampening of the primary effects of fatigue. Like Paroxetine, their use to treat fatigue in the absence of depression has not been formally assessed. Due to their propensity to cause increased confusion, use of tricyclic antidepressants in patients with cognitive impairment must be handled carefully, and routine use in this population is not typically recommended.

Atomoxetine is an agent that has also been promoted as a medication for arousal. Although most clinicians would associate this medication with the traditional neurostimulants, it is more similar pharmacologically to antidepressant drugs. Although no study has been conducted to evaluate its effects as a treatment for combating fatigue, anecdotal reports suggest that it may have a beneficial effect at higher doses.[60]

In patients with fatigue complicated by depression, the nature of their symptoms should be taken into account when choosing an appropriate treatment. When 1 symptom predominates, management should be tailored to treat that symptom along with the depression. For example, Trazodone can help with sleep initiation as seen with depression, whereas stimulants would be appropriate when fatigue or impaired concentration predominates.

Recent research has focused on endocrine abnormalities, especially growth hormone deficiency, as a potential cause for fatigue following TBI. However, the research has had mixed results. To date, a controlled study evaluating the effects of growth hormone replacement therapy on fatigue has not been completed. There is also some evidence that men with PD may have testosterone deficiency, though a study in 2006 that looked at testosterone therapy in this population found that the intervention had no effect on sleep or fatigue.[61]

Many herbal preparations have been promoted for use in fatigue. Among these are Ginkgo biloba, St. John's wort, and Panax ginseng. Although there is mounting anecdotal evidence that these herbal preparations are helpful in fatigue, there is no clear evidence. Caffeine, also considered a herbal remedy due to its widespread over-the-counter use, has been promoted as an agent to combat fatigue, both in its typical liquid form and as a tablet. Although caffeine is a potent stimulant, it can also cause unwanted side effects, such as anxiety and difficulty sleeping, so its recommended use should be in moderation only.

Nonpharmacologic Interventions

Although there is little literature on its efficacy, patient and caregiver education has become perhaps the most important rehabilitation intervention we have for combating fatigue. Patients should be educated on the underlying causes of fatigue and their potential impact and then be taught practical strategies to minimize and manage their symptoms (See **Table 4**.) This will give patients a sense of control and help diminish their frustration. Cognitive-behavioral therapy, which is based on teaching patients how to manage thoughts and behaviors, has been successful in decreasing fatigue as well.

Table 4
Behavioral modifications to minimize fatigue

1. Take frequent rests
2. Schedule breaks
3. Break up tasks
4. Avoid multitasking
5. Prioritize tasks
6. Delegate tasks
7. Focus on completing tasks rather than completing tasks quickly
8. Sleep hygiene strategies
9. Know side effects of medications
10. Do not operate heavy equipment or drive when fatigued
11. Recognize warning signs of fatigue
    a. Irritability
    b. Making mistakes
12. Custom-designed exercise protocol (when appropriate)

Post-stroke fatigue has significant impact on psychological and social functioning. A Polish study investigating the psychological aspects of stroke patients with fatigue showed that the patient's style of coping with stress can be predictive of fatigue.[62] Specifically, patients who use emotional-style coping showed a lower level of fatigue than did those who used task-oriented coping. This concept has implications for the development of psychologically based therapies focused on stress management.

Some traditional osteopathic techniques can also help treat fatigue in the neurologic population. One of the 4 central principles of osteopathic philosophy is that structure and function are reciprocally inter-related.[63] After a neurologic event such as a stroke, however, the function of key structures often becomes impaired, increasing the energy requirements for ADLs and the fatigue burden on a patient. Osteopathic physicians can employ various techniques to restore alignment and function, which may decrease the energy costs associated with normal activities, thus decreasing fatigue. There are also cranial manipulation techniques that have been successful anecdotally in decreasing fatigue and improving arousal.

Exercise training is another promising strategy for decreasing both physical and cognitive fatigue in persons with neurologic disorders. Because fatigue will intuitively diminish the amount of daily physical activity a person will engage in, it can hasten deconditioning and promote a further decrease in exercise tolerance. Onset of this cycle is a risk encountered by patients after the structured phase of their rehabilitation has ended. Patients should be educated as to the benefits of exercise and what precautions they should adhere to. Several studies have shown that a modest cardiovascular exercise routine can decrease overall fatigue in patients with PD. As with MS and diseases of the neuromuscular junction, patients and therapists should be cautioned not to exercise to the point of exhaustion, as this may have a paradoxical effect and actually increase overall fatigue. Emphasis should be on maintenance of function while decreasing general debility. Maximizing passive and active range of motion is critical to any muscular fitness program, and programs should be tailored to the appropriate neurologic and functional deficits at hand.

Aerobic exercise is well known to improve cognition, mood, and QoL in the general population. Cognitive functioning demonstrated improvement on neuropsychological tests for those individuals who were aerobically trained, compared with that of those who received strength and flexibility training as well as with that of those who did not exercise. Although research examining the effects of aerobic exercise on individuals with TBI, stroke, and PD is limited, exercise has been shown to be effective in improving cognition and depression in individuals with cancer, MS, fibromyalgia, dementia, chronic fatigue syndrome, and chronic obstructive pulmonary disease. In addition, studies have found aquatic therapy to result in strength gains. The gravity-eliminating conditions are beneficial to patients with neurologic weakness as well as many musculoskeletal conditions.

SUMMARY

Fatigue is a serious, QoL-limiting symptom of many neurologic conditions. Physicians should be thorough and consistent in their assessment for this problem and not let motor symptoms monopolize an office visit. Although the use of pharmacology to treat this problem has predominantly only anecdotal evidence of efficacy, several nonpharmacologic interventions may prove helpful. The directions of future research should aim to create clear treatment guidelines using the pharmacologic agents available.

REFERENCES

1. Zesiewica TA, Patel-Larsen A, Hauser RA, et al. Social Security Disability Insurance (SSDI) in Parkinson's disease. Disabil Rehabil 2007;29(24):1934–6.
2. Lou JS, Kearns G, Oken B, et al. Exacerbated physical fatigue and mental fatigue in Parkinson's disease. Mov Disord 2001;16(2):190–6.
3. Chaudhuri A, Behan PO. Fatigue and basal ganglia. J Neurol Sci 2000;179(S 1-2): 34–42.
4. Friedman J, Friedman H. Fatigue in Parkinson's disease. Neurology 1993;43: 2016–8.
5. van Hilten JJ, Weggeman M, van der Velde EA, et al. Sleep, excessive daytime sleepiness and fatigue in Parkinson's disease. J Neural Transm 1993;5:235–44.
6. Shulman LM, Taback RL, Bean J, et al. Comorbidity of the nonmotor symptoms of Parkinson's disease. Mov Disord 2001;16(3):507–10.
7. Karlsen K, Laresen JP, Tandberg E, et al. Fatigue in patients with Parkinson's disease. Mov Disord 1999;14(2):237–41.
8. Alves G, Wentzel-Larsen T, Larsen JP. Is fatigue an independent and persistent symptom in patients with Parkinson's disease? Neurology 2004;63(10): 1908–11.
9. De Groot MH, Phillips SJ, Eskes GA. Fatigue associated with stroke and other neurological conditions: implications for stroke rehabilitation. Arch Phys Med Rehabil 2003;84:1714–20.
10. Ingles JL, Eskes GA, Phillips SJ. Fatigue after stroke. Arch Phys Med Rehabil 1999;80:173–8.
11. Schepers VP, Visser-Meily AM, Ketelaar M, et al. Post-stroke fatigue: course and its relation to personal and stroke-related factors. Arch Phys Med Rehabil 2006; 87(2):184–8.
12. Kreutzer JS, Seel RT, Gourley E. The prevalence and symptom rates of depression after traumatic brain injury: a comprehensive examination. Brain Inj 2001; 15:563–76.
13. Szymanski HC, Linn R. A review of the postconcussion syndrome. Int J Psychiatry Med 1992;22:357–75.
14. Ouellet MC, Beaulieu- Bonneau S, Morin CM. Insomnia in patients with traumatic brain injury: frequency, characteristics and risk factors. J Head Trauma Rehabil 2006;21:199–212.
15. Ziino C, Ponsford J. Selective attention deficits and subjective fatigue following traumatic brain injury. Neuropsychology 2006;20:383–90.
16. Ziino C, Ponsford J. Vigilance and fatigue following traumatic brain injury. J Int Neuropsychol Soc 2006;12:100–10.
17. Azouvi P, Couillet J, Leclercq M, et al. Divided attention and mental effort after severe traumatic brain injury. Neuropsychologia 2004;42:1260–8.
18. Ouellet MC, Morin CM. Fatigue following traumatic brain injury: frequency, characteristics and associated factors. Rehabil Psychol 2006;51:140–9.
19. LaChapelle DL, Finlayson MA. An evaluation of subjective and objective measures of fatigue in patients with brain injury and healthy controls. Brain Inj 1998;12:649–59.
20. Olver JH, Ponsford JL, Curran CA. Outcome following TBI: a comparison between 2 and 5 years post-injury. Brain Inj 1996;10:841–8.
21. Borgaro SR, Baker J, Wethe JV, et al. Subjective reports of fatigue during early recovery from traumatic brain injury. J Head Trauma Rehabil 2005; 5:416–25.

22. Bushnik T, Englander J, Wright J. Patterns of fatigue and its correlates over the first 2 years after traumatic brain injury. J Head Trauma Rehabil 2008;23:25–32.

23. Rahman S, Griffin HJ, Quinn NP, et al. Quality of Life in Parkinson's disease: the relative importance of the symptoms. Mov Disord 2008;23(10):1428–34.

24. Havlikova E, et al. Impact of fatigue on quality of life in patients with Parkinson's disease. Eur J Neurol 2008;15(5):475–80.

25. Herlofson K, Larsen JP. The influence of fatigue on health-related quality of life in patients with Parkinson's disease. Acta Neurol Scand 2003;107(1):1–6.

26. van de Port IG, Kwakkel G, Schepers VP, et al. Is fatigue an independent factor associated with activities of daily living, instrumental activities of daily living and health-related quality of life in chronic stroke? Cerebrovasc Dis 2007;23(1):40–5.

27. Naess H, Waje-Andreassen U, Thomassen L, et al. Health-related quality of life among young adults with ischemic stroke on long-term follow-up. Stroke 2006; 37(5):1232–6.

28. van de Port IG, Klwakkel G, van Wijk I, et al. Susceptibility to deterioration of mobility long-term after stroke: a prospective cohort study. Stroke 2006;37(1):167–71.

29. Michael KM, Allen JK, Macko RF. Fatigue after stroke: relationship to mobility, fitness, ambulatory activity, social support, and falls efficacy. Rehabil Nurs 2006;31(5):210–7.

30. Michael K, Macko RF. Ambulatory activity intensity profiles, fitness, and fatigue in chronic stroke. Top Stroke Rehabil 2007;14(2):5–12.

31. Cantor JB, Ashman T, Gordon W, et al. Fatigue after traumatic brain injury and its impact on participation and quality of life. J Head Trauma Rehabil 2008;23:41–51.

32. Culbertson WC, Moberg PJ, Duda JE, et al. Assessing the executive function deficits of patients with PD: utility of the Tower of London-Drexel. Assessment 2004;11:27–39.

33. Bushnik T, Englander J, Katznelson L. Fatigue after TBI: association with neuro-endocrine abnormalities. Brain Inj 2007;21(6):559–66.

34. Kelly DF, McArthur DL, Levin H, et al. Neurobehavioral and quality of life changes associated with growth hormone insufficiency after complicated mild, moderate, or severe traumatic brain injury. J Neurotrauma 2006;23(6):928–42.

35. Uc EY, Rizzo M, Anderson SW, et al. Driving with distraction in Parkinson disease. Neurology 2006;67(10):1774–80.

36. Meindorfner C, Korner Y, Moller JC, et al. Driving in Parkinson's disease: mobility, accidents, and sudden onset of sleep at the wheel. Mov Disord 2005;20(7): 832–42.

37. Zesiewicz TA, Sullivan KL, Hauser RA. Nonmotor symptoms of Parkinson's disease. Expert Rev Neurother 2006;6(12):1811–22.

38. Borek LL, Amick MM, Friedman JH. Non-motor aspects of Parkinson's disease. CNS Spectr 2006;11(7):541–54.

39. Rochester L, Hetherington V, Jones D, et al. Attending to the task: interference effects of functional tasks on walking in Parkinson's disease and the roles of cognition, depression, fatigue, and balance. Arch Phys Med Rehabil 2004; 85(10):1578–85.

40. Garber CE, Friedman JH. Effects of fatigue on physical activity and function in patients with Parkinson's disease. Neurology 2003;60(7):1119–24.

41. Rochester L, Jones D, Hetherington V, et al. Gait and gait-related activities and fatigue in Parkinson's disease: what is the relationship? Disabil Rehabil 2006; 28(22):1365–71.

42. Lynch J, Mead G, Greig C, et al. Fatigue after stroke: the development and evaluation of a case definition. J Psychosom Res 2007;63(5):539–44.

43. Carlsson GE, Moller A, Blomstrand C. Consequences of mild stroke in persons <75 years—a 1-year follow-up. Cerebrovasc Dis 2003;16(4):383–8.
44. Carlsson GE, Moller A, Blomstrand C. A qualitative study of the consequences of 'hidden dysfunctions' one year after a mild stroke in persons <75 years. Disabil Rehabil 2004;26(23):1373–80.
45. Fichtenberg NL, Zafonte RD, Putnam S, et al. Insomnia in a post-acute brain injury sample. Brain Inj 2002;16:197–206.
46. Mahmood O, Rapport LJ, Hanks RA, et al. Neuropsychological performance and sleep disturbance following traumatic brain injury. J Head Trauma Rehabil 2004; 19:378–90.
47. Mead G, Lynch J, Greig C, et al. Evaluation of fatigue scales in stroke patients. Stroke 2007;38(7):2090–5.
48. Buck D, Jacoby A, Massey A, et al. Development and validation of NEWSQOL, the Newcastle Stroke-Specific Qualify of Life Measure. Cerebrovasc Dis 2004; 17(2-3):143–52.
49. Belza BL, Henke CJ, Yelin EH, et al. Correlation of fatigue in older adults with rheumatoid arthritis. Nurse Res 1993;42:93–9.
50. Lee H, Kim SW, Kim JM, et al. Comparing effects of methylphenidate, sertraline and placebo on neuropsychiatric sequelae in patients with traumatic brain injury. Hum Psychopharmacol 2005;20(2):97–104.
51. Mendonca DA, Menezes K, Jog MS. Methylphenidate improves fatigue scores in Parkinson disease: a randomized controlled trial. Mov Disord 2007;22(14):2070–6.
52. Nutt JG, Carter JH, Carlson NE. Effects of methylphenidate on response to oral levodopa: a double-blind clinical trial. Arch Neurol 2007;64(3):319–23.
53. Jha A, Weintraub A, Allshouse A, et al. A Randomized trial of Modafinil for the treatment of fatigue and excessive daytime sleepiness in individuals with chronic traumatic brain injury. J Head Trauma Rehabil 2008;23(1):52–63.
54. Ondo WG, Fayle R, Atassi F, et al. Modafinil for daytime somnolence in Parkinson's disease: double blind, placebo controlled parallel trial. J Neurol Neurosurg Psychiatr 2005;76(12):1636–9.
55. Pucci E, Branãs P, D'Amico R, et al. Amantadine for fatigue in multiple sclerosis. Cochrane Database Syst Rev 2007 Jan 24;(1):CD002818.
56. Oved D, Ziv I, Treves TA, et al. Effect of dopamine agonists on fatigue and somnolence in Parkinson's disease. Mov disord 2006;21(8):1257–61.
57. Leone H, Polsonetti BW. Amantadine for traumatic brain injury: does it improve cognition and reduce agitation? J Clin Pharm Ther 2005;30:101–4.
58. Lou JS, Kearns G, Benice T, et al. Levodopa improves physical fatigue in Parkinson's disease: a double-blind, placebo-controlled, crossover study. Mov Disord 2003;18(10):1108–14.
59. Choi-Kwon S, Choi J, Kwon SU, et al. Fluoxetine is not effective in the treatment of post-stroke fatigue: a double-blind, placebo-controlled study. Cerebrovasc Dis 2007;23(2-3):103–8.
60. Ripley DL. Atomoxetine for individuals with traumatic brain injury. J Head Trauma Rehabil 2006;21(1):85–8.
61. Okun MS, Fernandez HH, Rodriguez RL, et al. Testosterone therapy in men with Parkinson disease: results of the TEST-PD Study. Arch Neurol 2006;63(5):729–35.
62. Jaracz K, Mielcarek L, Kozubski W. Clinical and psychological correlates of post-stroke fatigue. Preliminary results. Neurol Neurochir Pol 2007;41(1):36–43.
63. Wells MR. Biomechanics: an osteopathic perspective. In: Ward RC, editor. Foundations for Osteopathic Medicine. Philadelphia: Lippincott Williams and Wilkins; 2003. p. 63–90.

Fatigue in Multiple Sclerosis

Anjali Shah, MD

KEYWORDS

- Multiple sclerosis • Fatigue • Neurorehabilitation • Human
- Quality of life • Treatment of fatigue

MS is a chronic, debilitating, inflammatory, and neurodegenerative disease of the CNS. There is no cure for the disease, and its management includes use of symptomatic agents and disease-modifying therapies to reduce and/or prevent relapses and disease progression. MS affects approximately 350,000 persons in the United States.[1,2] Its estimated prevalence is 1/1000 individuals in North America, and it is one of the most common causes of disability in young adults.

The symptoms of MS are numerous and include weakness, paresthesias, visual changes, spasticity, cognitive dysfunction, ataxia, and fatigue. Fatigue remains one of the most common and debilitating symptoms in MS and is quoted as one of the single most disabling symptoms.[3] Forty percent of MS patients state fatigue as their most disabling symptom.[4] It has been reported to cause profound disruption of quality of life in MS patients.[5] Approximately 20% of patients evaluated in primary care clinics experience fatigue.[6] In contrast, 96% of MS patients experience fatigue, 88% of whom report fatigue as a moderate to high problem.[5,7]

DEFINITION

There is no universally accepted definition of fatigue in MS patients. One common definition describes a "subjective lack of physical and/or mental energy, perceived by the individual or caregiver to interfere with usual and desired activities." Some other definitions include "pathologic exhaustion," "reversible motor and cognitive impairment with reduced motivation and desire to rest," and "difficulty with initiation of or sustaining voluntary activities that does not correlate with muscle weakness, depression, or muscle fatigue." Researchers in the United Kingdom interviewed MS patients first in face-to-face interviews and then using a questionnaire format to learn about patients' perceptions of fatigue. Patients described fatigue as a "reversible motor and cognitive impairment, with reduced motivation and desire to rest."[8]

Conflict of Interest: The author is a paid consultant for Biogen Idec, EMD Serono, and Teva Pharmaceuticals.
Department of Physical Medicine and Rehabilitation, University of Texas Southwestern Medical Center, 5323 Harry Hines Blvd, Mail Code 9055, Dallas, TX 75390-9055, USA
E-mail address: anjali.shah@utsouthwestern.edu

Phys Med Rehabil Clin N Am 20 (2009) 363–372
doi:10.1016/j.pmr.2008.12.003

It is important to differentiate between peripheral and central fatigue, as each has a unique etiology and treatment recommendation. Peripheral fatigue equates to muscle fatigue due to physical exertion and is alleviated with rest and associated with fatigability. Fatigue differs from fatigability, which is a generalized sense of exhaustion, not present at rest, affecting the patient after a few minutes of physical activity, and alleviated with rest. Central fatigue is much more subjective and is associated with difficulty with arousal and attention. The subject reports a feeling of constant exhaustion, which can lead to worsening vision or function. MS patients experience both central and peripheral fatigue. Therefore, differentiation between both types is vital to proper management.

IMPACT OF FATIGUE

Fatigue in the MS patient can have profound negative effects. Patients frequently need to nap, take frequent breaks, or sleep early. This may interfere with family activities, cause avoidance of the outdoors due to fatiguing effects of heat, or lead to an inability to participate in events that require prolonged physical effort. Social activities with friends and family are difficult to plan, as some days MS patients may awaken with an overwhelming sense of fatigue that cannot be alleviated with rest.[9] Cognitive processing, memory, and concentration are impaired during periods of fatigue.[10] Fatigue can negatively affect vocational performance and maintenance, especially if workplace accommodations are not achievable. The presence of fatigue has significant negative implications on quality of life in MS patients. Interestingly, as disease progresses, the effect of fatigue in MS frequently diminishes due to overall decreased ability of persons to perform previous routine activities.

MS patients often avoid physical activity to avoid fatigue. Additionally, patients may be concerned about thermosensitivity secondary to elevated body temperatures. Therefore, many MS patients engage in minimal physical activity, which may progressively worsen their weakness, fatigue, and other health issues. Limited mobility can play a role in worsening spasticity, constipation, and bone loss. In exercise studies, people with MS were shown to have decreased peak oxygen levels during maximal incremental exercise compared with those of healthy subjects.[11] This finding may suggest that MS patients have reduced cardiovascular fitness related to deconditioning. Insufficient activity in MS patients is linked to muscle changes that occur independently of CNS damage (ie, lowered oxidative capacity, lowered muscle dynamic properties, increased muscle fatigue, impaired metabolic responses to muscles to load, impaired excitation–contraction coupling).[12] Therefore, there may be an imbalance between the increased metabolic need in MS patients and their lowered cardiovascular supply. Rampello and colleagues[11] found that maximum exercise tolerance improved after patients completed 8 weeks of aerobic training, with a significant change in walking capacity. Similar results occurred after a 4-week aerobic treadmill training in MS patients with no worsening of fatigue scores.[13] Several studies have demonstrated clear benefit of regular physical activity in MS patients with improved fitness levels and quality-of-life measures.[6,11,12,14,15] However, not all results are linked with corresponding decreases in fatigue; conversely, no worsening of fatigue was reported.

In addition to the effect on health, personal life, and vocation, the costs of MS should be considered. Unexpectedly, healthcare costs increase with increasing disability.[16,17] The MS patient is responsible for the majority of the financial burden. The proportion of costs directly attributable to fatigue is unknown.

ASSESSMENT TOOLS

The Fatigue Severity Score (FSS), the Fatigue Impact Scale (FIS), and the Modified Fatigue Impact Scale (MFIS) are the most commonly used scales for fatigue assessment in MS patients.[18] The FSS is composed of 9 items that assess perceived fatigue.[19] Subjects are asked to assign a number from 1 (strongly disagree) to 7 (strongly agree) stating their agreement with each statement.[4] Responses are summed and averaged, with a score of 4 or more indicating significant fatigue.[20]

The FIS has been identified by the Multiple Sclerosis Council for Clinical Practice Guidelines "as the most appropriate for assessing the impact of MS-related fatigue on quality of life."[21] The FIS is a retrospective tool designed to evaluate fatigue during the past month. The FIS has separate subscales for physical, psychosocial, and cognitive functions, which span more than 40 statements.[9] Subjects are asked to score the effect of fatigue on those 4 dimensions using a 5-point scale from 0 (no problem) to 4 (extreme problem). Since the FIS takes approximately 10 to 20 minutes to be administered, followed by 5 minutes to score, shorter versions of the scale have been created. The MFIS is a modified version of the FIS and consists of a long (21-question) and short (5-question) version.[22] The total time to administer and score is about 10 to 15 minutes.

Kos and colleagues[22] developed a Visual Analog Scale that assesses the impact of fatigue on daily life, and they reported reliability and validity comparable to the FSS and MFIS. A score of 59 or more on a 100-mm line signifies individuals with fatigue that has a high impact on daily life. This may be helpful for the clinician to quickly assess fatigue in patients in the context of an office visit.

Although several scales are available for evaluation of fatigue in MS patients, none of them is an objective scale. All currently available scales are self-report questionnaires or surveys. Due to the fluctuating nature of MS, it is possible that patient's perception of fatigue is highly dependent on the time of day the survey was performed. A study evaluating walking parameters and fatigue in MS patients reported no significant difference in walking speed, stride length, cadence, or double-limb support time from 10 AM to 3 PM on the same day, whereas the self-reported fatigue score increased significantly.[23] This study is supported by findings from Krupp and colleagues[4] who found no relation between neurologic disability level and fatigue. This finding supports the need for objective measures in evaluating fatigue. However, the challenge in measuring the biological impact of fatigue is that the mechanisms of fatigue are largely unknown.

PATHOGENESIS—PRIMARY FACTORS

When evaluating the pathogenesis of fatigue in MS, it is important to distinguish primary fatigue from secondary fatigue. Primary fatigue is a result of the disease process, and secondary fatigue results from medications or disease-related manifestations.[24] Due to the multimodal aspect of fatigue in MS, it is difficult to differentiate primary fatigue from secondary fatigue, as several factors contribute to fatigue manifestation.

There are several theories on the pathogenesis of fatigue, with strong evidence for an inflammation mediated process. Giovannoni[7] and Heesen and colleagues[25] state that fatigue is inflammation driven, citing that fatigue caused by viral or bacterial infections can be reproduced by proinflammatory cytokines, such as interferon α or β or interleukin-2. Several MS patients experience fatigue as a side effect of interferon treatment. The potential effect of hypothalamo-pituitary-adrenal (HPA) axis dysfunction on fatigue has been evaluated by multiple researchers with varying results. HPA hypoactivity occurs in chronic fatigue syndrome, and researchers have searched for a connection with MS and fatigue. Some studies report no correlation between fatigue scores and abnormal dexamethasone–corticotropin-releasing hormone scores, whereas others report hyperactivity of the HPA axis.[26] Gadolinium (Gd) enhancing lesions, the quintessential marker for inflammation in MS, failed to demonstrate correlation between fatigue and Gd-enhancing lesions.

Some aspects of fatigue suggest that it may be related to underlying demyelinating pathology, which results in slowing and desynchronization of nerve transmission or partial or complete conduction block.[6,27] The peripheral causes of fatigue have been investigated using repetitive nerve stimulation (RNS). RNS failed to demonstrate improved impulse conduction along demyelinated nerves. Finally, central motor conduction time is prolonged in MS patients, supporting the use of evoked potential testing in MS patients for diagnostic purposes.

Some researchers correlate hypometabolism detected in positron emission tomography in the bilateral prefrontal cortex, premotor and supplemental motor cortex, putamen, and white matter extending from rostral putamen to the head of the caudate nucleus, with fatigue symptoms.[6,28] Diffuse axonal damage and brain atrophy are also linked as possibly related to causing fatigue.[29,30] No correlation between brain atrophy and fatigue has been found.[31,32] Functional magnetic resonance imaging displays impaired interaction between cortical and subcortical areas, which is inversely related to results on the FSS.

Researchers have raised the question whether MS fatigue is more of a peripheral than central phenomenon.[5] The hallmark of peripheral fatigue is muscle fatigability, frequently due to neuromuscular or myopathic disorders.[6] Sustained muscle fatigue leads to disuse atrophy, thereby limiting endurance in MS patients. This can lead to cardiovascular decline, increased spasticity, contracture development, and overall deconditioning. Central fatigue is characterized by a feeling of constant exhaustion and is associated with several neurologic disorders, including MS. Central fatigue is implicated in MS due to the correlation between fatigue and cognitive dysfunction.

PATHOGENESIS—SECONDARY FACTORS

There are several additional factors that may worsen fatigue for patients with MS (**Box 1**). Thermosensitivity is common in people with MS, leading to instability and delay in signal conduction in demyelinated nerves. Increased body temperature induces conduction block, resulting in deterioration of neurologic function, which is known as the Uhthoff phenomenon. MS fatigue secondary to heat sensitivity differs from that in normal healthy adults (NHAs) in that heat intolerance causes difficulty in sustaining physical activities and interferes with physical functions and responsibilities.[4] MS patients should be encouraged to precool with ice water or sit in a cool bath for 20 minutes before engaging in exercise or other forms of physical activity.[33]

Mood disorders, such as depression and anxiety, are common in MS patients. Depression occurs in approximately 50% of MS patients.[18] It may either occur as a secondary reaction to living with a chronic, debilitating condition, or it may be embedded in a mood disorder such as bipolar disease. Treatment with the serotonin reuptake inhibitor, fluoxetine, in combination with 4-aminopyridine (4-AP), has demonstrated reduced levels of fatigue in MS patients. A link between fatigue and psychiatric illness, most commonly depression, has been suggested. The results are mixed, with some reports finding no correlation and some finding strong correlation between psychiatric illness and MS fatigue.[34–37] Many researchers strongly support the fact that timely identification and management of mood disorders are vital. Psychiatric illnesses are rarely the sole cause of fatigue.

Box 1
Fatigue—secondary factors

Thermosensitivity

Depression

Anxiety

Sleep disturbance

Infection

    Viral

    Bacterial

Thyroid dysfunction

Anemia

Medications

    Antidepressants

    Antispasmodics

    Narcotics

    Sedatives

Many MS patients with fatigue also complain of sleep disturbance. This may be secondary to neuropathic pain, spasticity, or periodic limb movements. Obstructive sleep apnea should be ruled out as a contributing factor to fatigue. A significant correlation has been reported between fatigue and disrupted sleep or abnormal sleep cycles in MS patients.[38] Additionally, a study compared the incidence among French Canadians of restless leg movement (RLM) in 200 MS patients, 100 patients with rheumatoid arthritis, and 100 NHAs. They reported that 37.5% of MS patients, 31% of RA patients, 16% of NHAs fulfilled criteria for RLM.[39] A smaller study of 25 MS patients compared to 25 normal healthy controls reported RLM in 36% of MS patients. In addition, MS patients had reduced sleep efficiency and increased awakenings on 8-hour polysomnography testing.[40] Studies in this area remain limited, and further research is needed to gain a better understanding of the underlying mechanisms associated with MS sleep disturbance and fatigue. Surveillance of sleep quality is recommended in MS patients with fatigue.

Other medical conditions can contribute to fatigue, and that should be evaluated. Infections, either viral or bacterial, and, most commonly, urinary tract infections or upper respiratory infections can adversely affect energy levels in MS patients and worsen other symptoms such as spasticity and pain. Evaluation and exclusion of thyroid, liver, and hematologic profile abnormalities are encouraged.

Several of the medications prescribed for symptomatic treatment in MS patients can worsen fatigue. The clinician is encouraged to regularly review patients' medication lists for potential offenders. This includes antispasticity agents, antiepileptics, narcotics, or sedatives. Patients may report increased fatigue secondary to interferon treatment. The use of nonsteroidal anti-inflammatory drugs, such as naproxen or ibuprofen, has demonstrated efficacy over acetaminophen and is encouraged before and after interferon injection for effective management of flu-like effects.[41]

TREATMENT OF FATIGUE
Prevention

After ruling out primary and/or secondary causes of fatigue and deciding on treatment, it is important that the clinician's approach to the treatment of fatigue be global, including pharmacologic and nonpharmacologic approaches. Nonpharmacologic approaches include local cooling devices, energy management strategies (spacing out activities, performing strenuous activities during periods of increased energy stores), behavioral/lifestyle modifications (good sleep hygiene, limiting alcohol intake, tobacco cessation), nutrition management, and rehabilitative interventions.

Rehabilitative Interventions

The effect of various neurorehabilitative interventions on fatigue has been investigated. Yoga and bicycling demonstrated reduced fatigue and improved quality of life in MS patients.[42] An aerobic treadmill training program designed for MS patients of varying degrees of disability, exercising at 55% to 85% of age-predicted maximum heart rate, did not worsen fatigue.[13] Mathiowetz and colleagues[43] developed an energy conservation protocol for MS patients based on a model designed by Packer that was created for patients living with chronic illness. The 6-week, 2 h/wk energy conservation course was taught to 79 MS patients with varying types and degrees of severity of MS and was found to reduce fatigue impact and increase self-efficacy and quality of life. The use of physical and occupational therapists is encouraged to help patients with assistive devices for activities of daily living (ADL), using correct body mechanics, and assist with planning and time management to optimize energy levels.

Medications

Several medications have been found to be beneficial for reducing the severity of fatigue. Acetyl-L-carnitine (ALC) is a cellular component with a vital role in energy metabolism. ALC has demonstrated effectiveness in fatigue reductions in many chronic fatigue syndrome patients and in cancer patients undergoing chemotherapy. It has also demonstrated decrease in fatigue in MS patients.[44] ALC is believed to have direct neurotransmitter action in the brain and may play a role in the excitatory and inhibitory pathways.[45]

Amantadine, a tricyclic amine, is more widely known for its antiviral effect. Its mechanism of action is not clear, though it has monoaminergic, cholinergic, and glutaminergic effects.[18] Typical dosage is about 200 mg/d and is well tolerated. It significantly reduced fatigue in a placebo-controlled trial in MS patients.[46] When amantadine was compared with supplemental ALC in a crossover trial, ALC demonstrated superior efficacy and tolerance to amantadine.[44] Side effects of amantadine include insomnia, ankle edema associated with livedo reticularis, and nervousness.[47]

Potassium channel blockers, such as 3,4-AP and 4-AP, improve synaptic transmission and increase muscle twitch tension.[32] Titration of the drug is recommended, with doses ranging from 5 mg daily to 20 mg three times a day. Both 3,4 and 4-AP have demonstrated improvement in fatigue, weakness, and ambulation.[48–50] Side effects include vertigo, anxiety, nausea, seizures, confusion, and loss of consciousness.[34]

The effect of aspirin (acetylsalicylic acid [ASA]) on fatigue has been studied in a small double-blind, placebo-controlled study revealing modest benefit when dosed at 650 mg twice a day.[51] ASA irreversibly inhibits cyclooxygenase and blocks prostaglandin E2 production. Its effect on fatigue is believed to involve the HPA axis. Larger, long-term studies are recommended to further evaluate the benefit–risk profile.

Modafinil is Food and Drug Administration approved for use in persons with narcolepsy, obstructive sleep apnea, and shift workers. It is a central a-adrenergic agonist, acting in brain areas to increase wakefulness and increasing frontal lobe cortical activity.[52] The dosage ranges from 100 to 400 mg/d, and it is recommended that it should not be given later than lunchtime to avoid symptoms of insomnia. It has demonstrated improvement in 1 study over placebo at 200 mg/day, but not at the 400 mg/d dosage.[53] Another rigorous study reported no benefit of modafinil over placebo.[54] Additional trials are warranted, as several patients report significant relief of fatigue with modafinil. Side effects of modafinil include nervousness, headache, and nausea.[50]

Prokarin is a histamine-caffeine combination in a transdermal cream. Histamine as a therapeutic agent has been used in the treatment of Bell palsy, vasculitis, and Meniere disease for several years.[55] A 12-week, double-blind, placebo-controlled study of Prokarin demonstrated reduction in the MFIS by 37%. Serum caffeine levels were similar in both groups; therefore, the authors conclude that the primary cause of fatigue decrease was not caffeine intake alone. The cream was well tolerated, and side effects included skin rash and diarrhea.[50] Calcium supplementation is recommended to avoid increased stiffness.

SUMMARY

In summary, MS-related fatigue can be a severe problem causing interference with home and vocational activities. There are multiple factors that can contribute to fatigue in MS, and it is important for the patient, family, and clinician to be aware of potential confounders that may worsen fatigue. Clearer understanding about the etiology of fatigue is necessary. Additional larger, randomized, clinical trials are needed to evaluate etiology, pathophysiology, and both pharmacologic and nonpharmacologic interventions. Given the varying nature of fatigue and the limited evidence that fatigue in MS patients is highly dependent on self-perceived scores, additional research into the effect of psychosocial and psychological interventions is recommended. A multidisciplinary approach to fatigue is encouraged when treatments are considered for maximum benefit.

ACKNOWLEDGMENT

The author thanks Dr. Ian B. Maitin for his editorial comments on the manuscript.

REFERENCES

1. Anderson DW, Ellenberg JH, Leventhal CM, et al. Revised estimate of the prevalence of multiple sclerosis in the United States. Ann Neurol 1992;31(3):333–6.
2. Hirtz D, Thurman DJ, Gwinn-Hardy K, et al. How common are the "common" neurologic disorders? Neurology 2007;68(5):326–37.
3. Kraft GH, Freal JE, Coryell JK. Disability, disease duration, and rehabilitation service needs in multiple sclerosis: patient perspectives. Arch Phys Med Rehabil 1986;67(3):164–8.
4. Krupp LB, Alvarez LA, LaRocca NG, et al. Fatigue in multiple sclerosis. Arch Neurol 1988;45(4):435–7.
5. Hemmett L, Holmes J, Barnes M, et al. What drives quality of life in multiple sclerosis? QJM 2004;97(10):671–6.
6. Chaudhuri A, Behan PO. Fatigue in neurological disorders. Lancet 2004; 363(9413):978–88.

7. Giovannoni G. Multiple sclerosis related fatigue. J Neurol Neurosurg Psychiatry 2006;77(1):2–3.
8. Mills RJ, Young CA. A medical definition of fatigue in multiple sclerosis. QJM 2008;101(1):49–60.
9. Fisk JD, Pontefract A, Ritvo PG, et al. The impact of fatigue on patients with multiple sclerosis. Can J Neurol Sci 1994;21(1):9–14.
10. Hubsky EP, Sears JH. Fatigue in multiple sclerosis: guidelines for nursing care. Rehabil Nurs 1992;17(4):176–80.
11. Rampello A, Franceschini M, Piepoli M, et al. Effect of aerobic training on walking capacity and maximal exercise tolerance in patients with multiple sclerosis: a randomized crossover controlled study. Phys Ther 2007;87(5):545–55 [discussion: 555–549].
12. Rasova K, Brandejsky P, Havrdova E, et al. Spiroergometric and spirometric parameters in patients with multiple sclerosis: are there any links between these parameters and fatigue, depression, neurological impairment, disability, handicap and quality of life in multiple sclerosis? Mult Scler 2005;11(2):213–21.
13. van den Berg M, Dawes H, Wade DT, et al. Treadmill training for individuals with multiple sclerosis: a pilot randomised trial. J Neurol Neurosurg Psychiatry 2006; 77(4):531–3.
14. Newman MA, Dawes H, van den Berg M, et al. Can aerobic treadmill training reduce the effort of walking and fatigue in people with multiple sclerosis: a pilot study. Mult Scler 2007;13(1):113–9.
15. Rasova K, Havrdova E, Brandejsky P, et al. Comparison of the influence of different rehabilitation programmes on clinical, spirometric and spiroergometric parameters in patients with multiple sclerosis. Mult Scler 2006;12(2):227–34.
16. Bourdette DN, Prochazka AV, Mitchell W, et al. Health care costs of veterans with multiple sclerosis: implications for the rehabilitation of MS. VA Multiple Sclerosis Rehabilitation Study Group. Arch Phys Med Rehabil 1993;74(1):26–31.
17. Whetten-Goldstein K, Sloan FA, Goldstein LB, et al. A comprehensive assessment of the cost of multiple sclerosis in the United States. Mult Scler 1998;4(5):419–25.
18. Lapierre Y, Hum S. Treating fatigue. Int MS J 2007;14(2):64–71.
19. Packer TL, Sauriol A, Brouwer B. Fatigue secondary to chronic illness: postpolio syndrome, chronic fatigue syndrome, and multiple sclerosis. Arch Phys Med Rehabil 1994;75(10):1122–6.
20. Egner A, Phillips VL, Vora R, et al. Depression, fatigue, and health-related quality of life among people with advanced multiple sclerosis: results from an exploratory telerehabilitation study. NeuroRehabilitation 2003;18(2):125–33.
21. Mathiowetz V. Test-retest reliability and convergent validity of the Fatigue Impact Scale for persons with multiple sclerosis. Am J Occup Ther 2003;57(4):389–95.
22. Kos D, Nagels G, D'Hooghe MB, et al. A rapid screening tool for fatigue impact in multiple sclerosis. BMC Neurol 2006;6:1–8.
23. Morris ME, Cantwell C, Vowels L, et al. Changes in gait and fatigue from morning to afternoon in people with multiple sclerosis. J Neurol Neurosurg Psychiatry 2002;72(3):361–5.
24. Bakshi R. Fatigue associated with multiple sclerosis: diagnosis, impact and management. Mult Scler 2003;9(3):219–27.
25. Heesen C, Nawrath L, Reich C, et al. Fatigue in multiple sclerosis: an example of cytokine mediated sickness behaviour? J Neurol Neurosurg Psychiatry 2006; 77(1):34–9.
26. Gottschalk M, Kumpfel T, Flachenecker P, et al. Fatigue and regulation of the hypothalamo-pituitary-adrenal axis in multiple sclerosis. Arch Neurol 2005;62(2):277–80.

27. Zwarts MJ, Bleijenberg G, van Engelen BG. Clinical neurophysiology of fatigue. Clin Neurophysiol 2008;119(1):2–10.
28. Roelcke U, Kappos L, Lechner-Scott J, et al. Reduced glucose metabolism in the frontal cortex and basal ganglia of multiple sclerosis patients with fatigue: a 18F-fluorodeoxyglucose positron emission tomography study. Neurology 1997;48(6):1566–71.
29. Marrie RA, Fisher E, Miller DM, et al. Association of fatigue and brain atrophy in multiple sclerosis. J Neurol Sci 2005;228(2):161–6.
30. Tartaglia MC, Narayanan S, Francis SJ, et al. The relationship between diffuse axonal damage and fatigue in multiple sclerosis. Arch Neurol 2004;61(2):201–7.
31. Bakshi R, Miletich RS, Henschel K, et al. Fatigue in multiple sclerosis: cross-sectional correlation with brain MRI findings in 71 patients. Neurology 1999; 53(5):1151–3.
32. Mainero C, Faroni J, Gasperini C, et al. Fatigue and magnetic resonance imaging activity in multiple sclerosis. J Neurol 1999;246(6):454–8.
33. White AT, Wilson TE, Davis SL, et al. Effect of precooling on physical performance in multiple sclerosis. Mult Scler 2000;6(3):176–80.
34. Romani A, Bergamaschi R, Candeloro E, et al. Fatigue in multiple sclerosis: multi-dimensional assessment and response to symptomatic treatment. Mult Scler 2004;10(4):462–8.
35. Schwartz CE, Coulthard-Morris L, Zeng Q. Psychosocial correlates of fatigue in multiple sclerosis. Arch Phys Med Rehabil 1996;77(2):165–70.
36. Johansson S, Ytterberg C, Gottberg K, et al. Use of health services in people with multiple sclerosis with and without fatigue. Mult Scler 2009;15:88–95.
37. Ytterberg C, Johansson S, Andersson M, et al. Variations in functioning and disability in multiple sclerosis. A two-year prospective study. J Neurol 2008; 255(7):967–73.
38. Attarian HP, Brown KM, Duntley SP, et al. The relationship of sleep disturbances and fatigue in multiple sclerosis. Arch Neurol 2004;61(4):525–8.
39. Auger C, Montplaisir J, Duquette P. Increased frequency of restless legs syndrome in a French-Canadian population with multiple sclerosis. Neurology 2005;65(10):1652–3.
40. Ferini-Strambi L, Filippi M, Martinelli V, et al. Nocturnal sleep study in multiple sclerosis: correlations with clinical and brain magnetic resonance imaging findings. J Neurol Sci 1994;125(2):194–7.
41. Leuschen MP, Filipi M, Healey K. A randomized open label study of pain medications (naproxen, acetaminophen and ibuprofen) for controlling side effects during initiation of IFN beta-1a therapy and during its ongoing use for relapsing-remitting multiple sclerosis. Mult Scler 2004;10(6):636–42.
42. Oken BS, Kishiyama S, Zajdel D, et al. Randomized controlled trial of yoga and exercise in multiple sclerosis. Neurology 2004;62(11):2058–64.
43. Mathiowetz V, Matuska KM, Murphy ME. Efficacy of an energy conservation course for persons with multiple sclerosis. Arch Phys Med Rehabil 2001;82(4):449–56.
44. Tomassini V, Pozzilli C, Onesti E, et al. Comparison of the effects of acetyl L-carnitine and amantadine for the treatment of fatigue in multiple sclerosis: results of a pilot, randomised, double-blind, crossover trial. J Neurol Sci 2004;218(1–2): 103–8.
45. Shug AL, Schmidt MJ, Golden GT, et al. The distribution and role of carnitine in the mammalian brain. Life Sci 1982;31(25):2869–74.
46. The Canadian MS Research Group. A randomized controlled trial of amantadine in fatigue associated with multiple sclerosis. Can J Neurol Sci 1987;14(3):273–8.

47. van Oosten BW, Truyen L, Barkhof F, et al. Choosing drug therapy for multiple sclerosis. An update. Drugs 1998;56(4):555–69.

48. Rossini PM, Pasqualetti P, Pozzilli C, et al. Fatigue in progressive multiple sclerosis: results of a randomized, double-blind, placebo-controlled, crossover trial of oral 4-aminopyridine. Mult Scler 2001;7(6):354–8.

49. Sheean GL, Murray NM, Rothwell JC, et al. An open-labelled clinical and electrophysiological study of 3,4 diaminopyridine in the treatment of fatigue in multiple sclerosis. Brain 1998;121(Pt 5):967–75.

50. Lee D, Newell R, Ziegler L, et al. Treatment of fatigue in multiple sclerosis: a systematic review of the literature. Int J Nurs Pract 2008;14(2):81–93.

51. Wingerchuk DM, Benarroch EE, O'Brien PC, et al. A randomized controlled crossover trial of aspirin for fatigue in multiple sclerosis. Neurology 2005;64(7):1267–9.

52. Pozzilli C, Prosperini L, Sbardella E, et al. Interferon after 10 years in patients with multiple sclerosis. Neurol Sci 2006;27(Suppl 5):S369–72.

53. Rammohan KW, Lynn DJ. Modafinil for fatigue in MS: a randomized placebo-controlled double-blind study. Neurology 2005;65(12):1139–43; author reply 1995–1997.

54. Stankoff B, Waubant E, Confavreux C, et al. Modafinil for fatigue in MS: a randomized placebo-controlled double-blind study. Neurology 2005;64(7):1139–43.

55. Gillson G, Richard TL, Smith RB, et al. A double-blind pilot study of the effect of Prokarin on fatigue in multiple sclerosis. Mult Scler 2002;8(1):30–5.

Fatigue in Rheumatologic Diseases

John C. Pan, MD[a], David N. Bressler, MD[a,b],*

KEYWORDS

- Fatigue • Fatigability • Rheumatoid arthritis
- Cognitive behavioral therapy • Fibromyalgia
- Chronic fatigue syndrome • Exercise

Fatigue is a universally shared experience and a significant component of rheumatologic diseases. The fact that rheumatologic patients experience fatigue that negatively affects their quality of life has been well documented. What is less clearly understood are the multifactorial physical and emotional mechanisms that contribute to this fatigue and, as a result, limit effective treatment strategies, which to date still remain mostly empiric. Fatigue is often rated by patients with rheumatologic disease as one of the key factors leading to decreased quality of life. Fatigue is poorly correlated with the severity of disease. Despite the omnipresence of and the stress caused by fatigue, it is surprising how infrequently it is addressed by both patients and physicians. Rheumatologic patients often believe that fatigue is an expected part of the disease process or a side effect of medications. Physicians, however, either dismiss the fatigue as functional in origin or focus more on joint and muscle involvement or abnormal laboratory values.

DEFINITION

There are many definitions of fatigue offered in the medical literature. However, for the purpose of discussing rheumatologic disease, a more global, biopsychosocial orientation is applied. As quoted in the *Physiologic Basis of Rehabilitation Medicine*,[1] Dill offered the following definition: "The various unmistakably disagreeable sensations commonly referred to the word fatigue are in fact the accompaniment of a great variety of physiologic conditions, which have in common only this, that the physiologic equilibrium of the body is breaking down." A distinction should also be made between

[a] Department of Rehabilitation Medicine, Mount Sinai School of Medicine, Mount Sinai Medical Center, One Gustave Levy Place, Box 1240, New York, NY 10029, USA
[b] Department of Rehabilitation Medicine, Elmhurst Hospital, 7901 Broadway, Elmhurst, NY 11373, USA
* Corresponding author. Attending Physiatrist, Department of Rehabilitation Medicine, Elmhurst Hospital, 7901 Broadway, Elmhurst, NY 11373, USA.
E-mail address: mandomolly357@yahoo.com (D.N. Bressler).

Phys Med Rehabil Clin N Am 20 (2009) 373–387
doi:10.1016/j.pmr.2008.12.008
1047-9651/08/$ – see front matter. Published by Elsevier Inc.

fatigue and fatigability, the latter being defined as progressive weakness of muscle with repetitive use followed by recovery after a brief period of rest. Fatigability has also remained underdiagnosed and may be an additional component of the global picture of fatigue in rheumatologic disorders.

Despite the pervasive and negative impact that fatigue can have on quality-of-life issues in the patient with rheumatologic disease, it does serve an important function as the body's "warning signal," forcing an individual to stop what he is doing and evaluate what is wrong.[2]

This article reviews fatigue as it occurs in 4 common rheumatologic disorders: fibromyalgia syndrome (FMS), chronic fatigue syndrome (CFS), rheumatoid arthritis (RA), and osteoarthritis (OA).

ASSESSMENT OF FATIGUE
History

Despite the significant negative impact fatigue imposes on the rheumatologic patient, it is often not addressed in clinical settings. Wolfe and Pincus reported that 89.7% of rheumatologists do not usually assess fatigue in their offices, and fewer than 15% collect any formal quantitative information regarding fatigue, psychological distress, and functional disability.[3] Patient self-report questionnaires have been found to be a valuable tool in assessing fatigue and monitoring functional status. Wolfe and colleagues[3,4] advocated the routine use of questionnaires as an integral part of patient care, which correlated with traditional measures, such as laboratory tests and radiographs. Moreover, questionnaires can be more effective in predicting long-term mortality and morbidity than measurements such as grip strength, walk time, or joint count. Multidimensional health status questionnaires such as Modified Health Assessment Questionnaire and Health Assessment Questionnaire (HAQ) have both been shown to be strong predictors of mortality in rheumatologic diseases. In 1 study involving 7760 patients, Wolfe showed that a single question asking patients to rate their fatigue in the past week on the visual analog scale (VAS) performed as well as 3 other significantly longer questionnaires. The single-item VAS fatigue scale was even more sensitive in detecting change in fatigue level than longer questionnaires.[5] To use patient questionnaire effectively, it should be administered to all patients attending the clinic on a sequential basis.

A large number of fatigue scales exist, and there is no consensus on which fatigue-measuring scales are most appropriate for use in assessment of fatigue in rheumatologic disease.[6] Fatigue is multidimensional in expression, with influence on physical, emotional, cognitive, and even social aspects of life. This created a challenge in its measurement. Many recent articles have focused on a questionnaire called functional assessment of chronic illness therapy (FACIT).[7] This instrument was initially employed to evaluate fatigue in anemia and cancer patients. Recent studies, however, have evaluated its efficacy in rheumatologic disease. The FACIT-fatigue is an abbreviated 13-item measure of fatigue that has showed good internal consistency in patients with RA when compared with other extensive scales (**Table 1**).

This scale is easy to administer, patient-friendly, and provides reliable insights into the causes of fatigue. It can be easily adapted to other rheumatologic diseases such as fibromyalgia and OA.[8]

Physical Examination

Fatigue is frequently not addressed in physical examinations during routine office visits, primarily due to its complex physiologic and psychosocial nature. To better

Table 1
FACIT-Fatigue Scale (Version 4)

Below is a list of statements that other people with your illness have said are important. Please circle or mark 1 number per line to indicate your response as it applies to the *past 7 days*

	Not at all	A little bit	Somewhat	Quite a bit	Very much
I feel fatigued.	0	1	2	3	4
I feel weak all over.	0	1	2	3	4
I feel listless ("washed out").	0	1	2	3	4
I feel tired.	0	1	2	3	4
I have trouble *starting* things because I am tired.	0	1	2	3	4
I have trouble *finishing* things because I am tired.	0	1	2	3	4
I have energy.	0	1	2	3	4
I am able to do my usual activities.	0	1	2	3	4
I need to sleep during the day.	0	1	2	3	4
I am too tired to eat.	0	1	2	3	4
I need help doing my usual activities.	0	1	2	3	4
I am frustrated by being too tired to do the things I want to do.	0	1	2	3	4
I have to limit my social activity because I am tired.	0	1	2	3	4

Reprinted with permission from David Cella, PhD. FACIT-Fatigue Scale. Functional assessment of chronic illness therapy website. Available at: http://www.facit.org/qview/qlist.aspx. Accessed October 7, 2008.

delineate the objective physical manifestation of fatigue, the term *fatigability* has been used, which is defined as diminished strength as exercise of muscle groups proceeds. Experimental studies that test for fatigability have employed dynamometer, electrical stimulation of peripheral nerves, and transcranial magnetic stimulations. In routine clinical settings, fatigability can be assessed by manual muscle testing after repetitive movement of functionally important muscles. Dobkin offered the following approach:[9]

The examiner could choose 10 to 15 repetitions of (1) raising the extended arms overhead or reaching and lifting an item, followed by retesting the strength of the isolated deltoids at 60° of abduction; (2) repetitive extension of the fingers against the modest resistance of an examiner's finger; (3) repetitive 30° hip flexor movements with the patient supine and leg extended at the knee followed by retesting strength of the iliopsoas at 20° of hip flexion; (4) repetitive 20° hip extensor movements against gravity or a modest force with the patient prone; (5) repetitive 60° knee flexor movements while prone against only gravity or modest resistance, followed by retesting the hamstrings with the knee flexed 30°, and so on. Retesting that reveals any decline from the initial torque and that resolves after a minute of rest would be consistent with exercise-induced fatigability.

Laboratory tests are not routinely used for the monitoring of fatigue, since fatigue has been found to correlate with pain and depression and not with disease activity as reflected by laboratory tests such as erythrocyte sedimentation rate or rheumatoid factor.[10]

FATIGUE IN FIBROMYALGIA

Perhaps no rheumatologic disorder is more associated with fatigue than FMS, the most common widespread pain disorder in the United States. Fibromyalgia affects 2% of 4% of the general population, and between 76% and 81% of people with fibromyalgia suffer from the symptom of chronic fatigue.[11,12] FMS is a syndrome without known pathologic agents, whose cardinal symptoms include pain, fatigue, and nonrestorative sleep. Specific criteria for the diagnosis of FMS were established in 1990 by the American College of Rheumatology (ACR) [**Table 2**].

Pain and Fatigue

Although a distinct cause for FMS is unknown, the most commonly accepted theories include the following: (1) central sensitization, with dysfunctional processing of pain by the central nervous system, (2) suppression of descending inhibitory pain pathways, (3) various neurohumoral dysregulations, especially those involving serotonin, norepinephrine, and substance P, (4) suppression and dysregulation of the hypothalamic-pituitary-adrenal axis.[13–17] Regardless of the pathologic mechanism(s), the result is widespread body pain, which, in turn, is closely associated with overwhelming fatigue. Common patient complaints often reflect this inter-relationship between pain and fatigue, for example, "The pain wears me down" or "When I'm tired I hurt all over." Fibromyalgia patients often describe the fatigue as overwhelming, exhaustive, debilitating, or incapacitating. Patients literally describe having to stop what they are doing and lie down. Wolfe and Pincus in a study in Rheumatology 1999 noted that in multivariate analysis, the strongest independent predictors for fatigue were pain, sleep disturbance, depression, tender point count, and HAQ.[3] In a 2007 study, pain was confirmed as among the strongest predictors of fatigue: "Individuals with higher average level of pain reported greater fatigue and daily increase in pain were related to daily increase in fatigue, including elevation of fatigue on the next day."[18] A 2008

Table 2
Criteria for the classification of fibromyalgia[66]

1. History of widespread pain

Definition. Pain is considered widespread when all of the following are present: pain in the left side of the body, pain in the right side of the body, pain above the waist, and pain below the waist. In addition, axial skeletal pain (cervical spine, anterior chest, thoracic spine, or low back) must be present. In the definition, shoulder and buttock pain is considered as pain for each involved side. "Low back" pain is considered lower segment pain.

2. Pain in 11 of 18 tender point sites on digital palpation

Definition. Pain, on digital palpation, must be present in at least 11 of the following 18 tender point sites:

- Occiput: bilateral, at the suboccipital muscle insertions
- Low cervical: bilateral, at the anterior aspects of the intertransverse spaces at C5–C7
- Trapezius: bilateral, at the midpoint of the upper border
- Supraspinatus: bilateral, at origins, above the scapula spine near the medial border
- Second rib: bilateral, at the second costochondral junctions, just lateral to the junctions on upper surfaces
- Lateral epicondyle: bilateral, 2 cm distal to the epicondyles
- Gluteal: bilateral, in upper outer quadrants of buttocks in anterior fold of muscle
- Greater trochanter: bilateral, posterior to the trochanteric prominence
- Knee: bilateral, at the medial fat pad proximal to the joint line

For classification purposes, patients will be said to have fibromyalgia if both criteria are satisfied. Widespread pain must have been present for at least 3 months. The presence of a second clinical disorder does not exclude the diagnosis of fibromyalgia. Digital palpation should be performed with an approximate force of 4 kg. For a tender point to be considered "positive," the subject must state that the palpation was painful. "Tender" is not to be considered "painful."

workshop sponsored by the National Institute of Aging noted that physical functioning in FMS, RA, and OA was predicted by pain and fatigue but not by pain alone.[2]

Nonrestorative Sleep and Fatigue

Nonrestorative, fragmented sleep is a constituent of the fibromyalgia syndrome and a significant contributor to the fatigue experienced by the fibromyalgia patient. Nearly all patients suffering from FMS experience poor sleep quality,[19] and the fatigue that follows is so pervasive that half of the patients who meet ACR criteria for FS also meet criteria for CFS.[20] Fibromyalgia patients were also reported to have higher stress responses to a variety of stimuli, which in turn compromise sleep and in turn exacerbate fatigue.[21,22]

Mental Fatigue ("Fibrofog")

Cognitive deficits involving memory and mental clarity referred to as "fibrofog" are common in FMS.[23–25] However, formal cognitive testing often does not support deterioration. FMS patients can experience dissociation or disengagement, which refers to the separation of parts of experience from the mainstream of consciousness. A common example is highway hypnosis.[23]

Evaluating Fatigue in Fibromyalgia

In evaluating fatigue in the fibromyalgia patient, there is a temptation to ascribe fatigue to the disease itself, rather than looking for alternative causes. Although no longer considered a diagnosis of exclusion, many conditions can mimic and occur concurrently with FMS and produce significant fatigue (**Table 3**).

| Table 3 |
Conditions that simulate fibromyalgia or occur concurrently with fibromyalgia[20]
Common
Hypothyroidism
Medications (especially lipid-lowering drugs, antiviral agents)
Polymyalgia rheumatica
Hepatitis C
Sleep apnea
Parvovirus infection
Cervical stenosis/Chiari malformation
Less common
Autoimmune disorders (eg, systemic lupus erythematosus, rheumatoid arthritis)
Endocrine disorders (eg, Addison disease, hyperparathyroidism)
Lyme disease
Eosinophilia-myalgia syndrome
Tapering of corticosteroids
Malignancy

Failure to identify another disease process responsible for the fatigue will significantly compromise both treatment and outcome. An initial laboratory analysis for patients who present with fatigue and have criteria consistent with FMS should include the following: complete blood count, urine analysis, erythrocyte sedimentation rate, and thyroid-stimulating hormone. Other tests such as antinuclear antibody, rheumatoid factor, serum complement levels, Lyme titers, Epstein-Barr virus test, muscle enzymes, radiographs, or other imaging studies are warranted only if the history and physical examination suggest a particular diagnosis.[20]

Treatment of Fatigue in Fibromyalgia

As described, the causes of fatigue in rheumatologic disease are multifactorial. Therefore, comprehensive treatment programs that incorporate pharmacologic and nonpharmacologic treatment strategies would appear to be the most efficacious.

Pharmacologic treatment of fatigue in FMS

Numerous medications, including serotonin specific reuptake inhibitors, serotonin-norepinephrine reuptake inhibitors, psychostimulants, and so on, have been employed in the management of fatigue. Four of the most currently prescribed medications are discussed. The tricyclics amitriptyline (Elavil) and cyclobenzaprine (Flexeril) have been considered mainstay agents in the management of FMS for many years. Although considered an antidepressant and muscle relaxant, respectively, both are structurally tricyclic compounds.

Amitriptyline A systematic Medline Cochrane review of amitriptyline in the management of FMS noted that at 25 mg a day, fatigue, in addition to pain and fragmented sleep, was improved but short lived. No positive effects were noted at 12 weeks. As such, the author stated, "A definitive clinical recommendation regarding the efficacy of amitriptyline for fibromyalgia symptoms cannot be made."[26]

Cyclobenzaprine A 2004 meta-analysis of the effectiveness of cyclobenzaprine noted no reduction in fatigue but some general overall improvement in well-being.[27]

Pregabalin (Lyrica) Approved by the FDA in June 2007, pregabalin is the first medication approved for the treatment of FMS. A 2008 randomized, double-blind, placebo-controlled study reported that pregabalin at 300, 450, and 600 mg a day was safe and effective in the treatment of fibromyalgia, but no significant improvement in fatigue was noted.[28] This lack of improvement in fatigue was felt to be due to pregabalin's side effect of daytime somnolence.[29]

Duloxetine (Cymbalta) Approved by the FDA in June 2008, duloxetine was the second medication approved for FMS. A 2008 study in *Pain* reported that duloxetine at 600 mg a day appears to be safe and efficacious in the treatment of FMS, with mental fatigue score improved at the end of the 6-month trial period.[30]

   A difficulty with many of these studies is that they evaluate the efficacy of a particular medication compared with placebo. What is lacking are studies comparing these medications to each other or comparing combinations of medications or combined pharmacologic and nonpharmacologic programs.

Cognitive-behavioral therapy for fatigue in FMS

Cognitive-behavioral therapy (CBT) is a stress inoculation training that involves the teaching of life and coping skills to minimize fatigue, pain, and stressful events.[31] A 2006 study compared the efficacy of CBT to pharmacologic intervention. The authors concluded that CBT was efficacious and must be considered a primary treatment in FMS.[32]

CHRONIC FATIGUE SYNDROME

CFS is a condition similar to, and often confused with, FMS. The overlap between these 2 syndromes is striking.[20] CFS has been described as a subset of FMS or as a distinct entity.[33] Women are diagnosed as having CFS 2 to 4 times as often as men, and the condition occurs most commonly in patients in their 40s and 50s.[34] The underlying pathophysiology of CFS is currently believed to be similar to that of FMS and includes atypical sensory processing in the central nervous system and dysfunction of skeletal muscle nociception and the hypothalamic-pituitary axis.[35] The specific diagnostic criteria for CFS are outlined in **Table 4**.[36]

   The hallmark of CFS is the presence of overwhelming fatigue of at least 6 months' duration that is not restored with rest. As outlined in **Table 4**, CFS also includes symptoms of sore throat, lower-grade fever, and lymph node tenderness, suggesting a possible viral etiology. Despite these findings, the specific cause(s) of CFS remain unclear. It should be noted that FMS patients may also complain of viral-like symptoms, making the distinction between CFS and FMS difficult. In fact, the 2 symptoms may overlap or even occur concurrently.

   Like FMS, there is no confirmatory laboratory test for CFS, and, therefore, the diagnosis rests exclusively on the patients presenting symptoms. Currently, there are no approved medications for the treatment of CFS. However, duloxetine is currently being investigated for the treatment of fatigue in CFS in a double-blind, randomized, control study in collaboration with its manufacturer, Eli Lilly. Study completion is scheduled for December 2009.[37] Trials of the psychostimulant modafinil (Provigil) have provided inconsistent results and, therefore, cannot be recommended for CFS.[38] CBT has been proven efficacious in reducing the symptoms of fatigue in CFS and may be more effective in reducing fatigue symptoms compared with other psychological therapies.[39] Like FMS, many research articles lend support to the effectiveness of CBT in the management of fatigue in CFS. The Cochrane Collaboration advises a *graded* exercise program for patients with CFS. Overstrenuous exercise

Table 4
1994 International Research Case Definition of Chronic Fatigue Syndrome[36]
CFS is a syndrome characterized by fatigue that is
Medically unexplained
Of new onset
Of at least 6 mo duration
Not the result of ongoing exertion
Not substantially relieved by rest
Causes a substantial reduction in previous levels of occupational, educational, social, or personal activities
In addition, there must be 4 or more of the following symptoms:
Impaired memory or concentration
Sore throat
Tender neck (cervical) or armpit (axillary) lymph nodes
Muscle pain (myalgia)
Headaches of a new type, pattern, or severity
Unrefreshing sleep
Postexertional malaise (lasting more than 24 h)
Multijoint pain (arthralgia without swelling or redness)
Conditions that would exclude a diagnosis of CFS include other medical disorders known to cause fatigue, major depressive illness, medications that cause fatigue as a side effect, and alcohol or substance abuse.

should be avoided, because it can exacerbate symptoms and promote immune system dysfunction.[40] The combination of graded exercise, CBT, which emphasizes *active* coping skills, paced daily activities, adequate rest, and a healthy life style appears to be the most efficacious and practical plan for managing CFS.

FATIGUE IN RHEUMATOID ARTHRITIS
Predictors of Fatigue in Rheumatoid Arthritis

Fatigue is a common symptom in RA, reported in 80% to 93% of individuals with RA, and can be perceived as the most problematic aspect of the disease.[41] In one study, pain and depressive symptoms were found to be the best predictors of fatigue in RA patients, whereas longer symptom duration, less perceived adequacy of social support, and less disease activity were also significant predictors of fatigue.[41] In another study comparing fatigue in RA, OA, and FMS, pain was found to be the strongest predictor of fatigue.[18] In a large study involving 24,831 patients, Wolfe and colleagues[42] concluded that pain, functional loss, depression, and sleep disturbance, and not inflammation, were the proximate causes of fatigue. Similar findings were also reported by Pollard and colleagues[10] in a cross-sectional study evaluating RA patients on anti-tumor necrosis factor (TNF) or disease-modifying antirheumatic drug (DMARD) treatment, which concluded that fatigue was associated with pain and changes in mental health, particularly depression, and not disease activity.

Treatment of Fatigue in Rheumatoid Arthritis

Improvement in fatigue as a consequence of effective treatment in pain has been widely reported. In a randomized controlled trial (RCT) involving 271 RA patients, Weinblatt and colleagues[43] showed that patients receiving Adalimumab, an anti-TNF antibody, plus methotrexate, had significantly less fatigue and pain than those in patients receiving placebo plus methotrexate. In an observational study with 30 patients receiving anti-TNF and 54 patients receiving DMARDs, Pollard and colleagues[10] showed that both treatments resulted in a decrease in fatigue, which correlated with improvement in pain. In an RCT by Cohen and colleagues, RA patients who had failed anti-TNF agents received rituximab plus methotrexate (n = 311) and had significantly less fatigue and better quality of life than patients receiving placebo plus methotrexate (n = 209).[44] Similar results with rituximab were also reported in other RCTs.[45,46] Chronic interpersonal stress is associated with greater stimulated cellular production of interleukin 6 along with impaired capacity of glucocorticoids to inhibit the cellular inflammatory response, leading to increased fatigue in RA patients.[47] Despite the apparent efficacy of TNF inhibitors in ameliorating fatigue, there are conflicting studies that do not support the positive studies noted here. Wolfe investigated 21,016 RA patients participating in the National Data Bank for Rheumatic Diseases and found that patients receiving anti-TNF therapy did not have lower fatigue scores compared with those of patients not treated with anti-TNF agents.[42] Therefore, the known efficacy of TNF inhibitor in the treatment of RA remains controversial when specifically applied to the treatment of fatigue.

OSTEOARTHRITIS

Fatigue in OA is not routinely evaluated. However, a growing number of studies have shown that fatigue is a crucial component of the disease.[48–50] Murphy and colleagues[48] measured ambulatory OA patients' physical activity by wrist-worn accelerometers and demonstrated that fatigue is strongly associated with physical inactivity in OA patients. Wolfe reported that OA patients had a similar level of fatigue as that of RA patients, and the 2 diseases shared the same predictors for fatigue: pain, depression, and functional loss.[5] In a qualitative study, Power and colleagues[51] also identified pain and depression as major factors in OA fatigue. Zautra and colleagues[18] noted that there are important differences between OA, RA, and FMS patients in both everyday manifestation and the bio-psychosocial correlates of fatigue. Fatigue in OA is influenced by daily pain fluctuation but to a lesser extent than that in RA or fibromyalgia.

EXERCISE
Exercise in Fibromyalgia

There is emerging evidence that exercise is beneficial in reducing fatigue in fibromyalgia. In a 2008 review article, the Ottawa Panel considered 13 RCTs and 3 controlled trials using aerobic fitness exercises for managing fibromyalgia. Grade A recommendations (based on RCT showing statistically significant clinical importance >15%) were given to aerobic exercise in relieving pain and depression, reducing VAS score for "lack of energy" by 30% and improving cardiopulmonary function, endurance, and positive affect. However, direct measurement of fatigue in 2 trials only received grade C recommendation (not statistically or clinically significant). In addition, the Ottawa Panel considered 5 RCTs using strengthening exercises in fibromyalgia and gave grade A recommendation for fatigue, depression, muscle strength, and short-term pain relief.[52,53] The article mentioned that most trials were rated low quality, but the panel still recommended the use of aerobic fitness as well as strengthening exercises based on the emerging evidence. A study involving postmenopausal women with FMS lends further support to the benefit of concurrent strength and endurance training in reducing fatigue in FMS. This study reinforces the concept that low-intensity strength training and aerobic exercises can decrease fatigue even though the amount of training was too low to improve general strength and not intensive enough to improve Vo_{2max}.[54]

Exercise in Chronic Fatigue Syndrome

The exercise program outlined for FMS is the same for CFS, which is a graded exercise program incorporating aerobic and strength training.

Exercise in Rheumatoid and Osteoarthritis

Exercise has been found to decrease fatigue in OA and RA. The Ottawa Panel Evidence-Based Clinical Practice Guidelines recommend the use of therapeutic exercises for OA after considering 26 RCTs.[55] Both strengthening exercises and general fitness exercises were recommended. The same panel also recommended whole-body, low-intensity exercises for RA patients based on 16 RCTs.[56] The Ottawa Panel used pain and function as outcomes and did not specifically address fatigue. However, knowing that pain, along with depression, is one of the strongest predictor of fatigue in OA and RA, it is reasonable to hypothesize that exercise significantly reduces fatigue. This result was confirmed in an RCT of 220 RA patients using low-impact, aerobic, group and home exercises, which showed that fatigue, pain, and depression decreased after 12 weeks of exercise.[57]

High- versus Low-Intensity Exercise for Rheumatoid Arthritis

For RA patients, traditionally, low-intensity, isometric, muscle strengthening, and range-of-motion exercises have been advocated. High-intensity, dynamic exercises were considered inappropriate because of fear of exacerbating inflammation and creating more joint damage.[56] However, current studies support the principle that high-intensity exercise is beneficial. An RCT with 281 patients in 2004 by de Jong and colleagues showed that patients receiving high-intensity, weight-bearing exercises actually developed less radiological damage during a 2-year period than that of patients not receiving such a structured exercise program.[58] In another RCT, van den Ende and colleagues[59] also showed that patients hospitalized because of an exacerbation of their disease did better with an intensive exercise program than patients performing a conservative program; no deleterious effects on disease activity were found. Similar results were also reported by other RCTs.[60,61]

An example of a high-intensity, 12-week outpatient exercise program for patients with well-controlled RA is as the following: Patients attend 1-hour group exercise sessions 3 times a week, which includes warming up, bicycling for 20 minutes, dynamic weight-bearing exercises such as knee bending, step-ups, walking at fast speed, and muscle strengthening for trunk and upper extremities. Every 4 weeks, patients are introduced to a new set of exercises with a higher exercise load. During bicycling, heart rate was maintained at 70% to 85% of the age-predicted maximum heart rate.[60]

Bracing, Energy Conservation, and Adaptive Equipment

There is some evidence that knee bracing in patients with unicompartmental OA reduces pain, improves gait, and reduces compartmental load.[62] Taping of the patella was also shown to produce clinically meaningful decrease in chronic OA knee pain.[63] For RA patients, a joint protection educational program that focuses on energy conservation techniques and adaptive equipments has been shown to reduce pain and improve activities of daily living.[64,65] These studies did not directly evaluate the effect of intervention on patient fatigue. However, recognizing that pain is one of the strongest predictors of fatigue, these interventions may empirically be beneficial in rheumatologic patients with significant fatigue.

SUMMARY

Today, fatigue still remains an under-reported symptom in rheumatologic diseases, infrequently addressed by patient and physician. Although not all of the causes of fatigue in rheumatologic diseases have been fully elucidated, recognizing the multifactorial components is essential in formulating targeted, effective treatment strategies. Deconstructing rheumatologic diseases into discrete symptoms such as fatigue in an effort to identify specific causes and formulate targeted treatments remains a daunting task. High-quality RCTs will be required to evaluate the effectiveness of combined pharmacologic and non-pharmacologic strategies, which empirically appear to be the most promising. To date, this research is lacking.

CLINICAL PEARLS

1. Always ask patient about fatigue—use VAS and short fatigue questionnaire.
2. Rule out nonrheumatologic causes of fatigue.
3. Identify and treat causative factors of fatigue, especially pain and depression.
4. Make the treatment individualized and multidimensional and inclusive of the following:
   - Appropriate medications (ie, duloxetine, pregabalin for FMS)
   - Combined aerobic exercise and strength training
   - CBT
5. Reassure the patient that significant improvement can occur over time with active participation and an effective treatment strategy.

REFERENCES

1. Gonzalez EG, Myers SJ, Edelstein JE, et al, editors. 3rd edition, Physiologic basis of rehabilitation medicine, vol. 16. Massachusetts: Butterworth Heinemann; 2004. p. 392.
2. Unexplained Fatigue in the Elderly—June 25–26, 2007 Workshop Summary. National Institute on Aging Website. Available at: http://www.nia.nih.gov/ResearchInformation/ConferencesAndMeetings/UnexplainedFatigue.htm. Updated April 17, 2008. Accessed August 21, 2008.
3. Wolfe F, Pincus T. Listening to the patient: a practical guide to self-report questionnaires in clinical care. Arthritis Rheum 1999;42(9):1797–808.
4. Wolfe F, Michaud K. Assessment of pain in rheumatoid arthritis: minimal clinically significant difference, predictors, and the effect of anti-tumor necrosis factor therapy. J Rheumatol 2007;34(8):1674–83.
5. Wolfe F. Fatigue assessments in rheumatoid arthritis: comparative performance of visual analog scales and longer fatigue questionnaires in 7760 patients. J Rheumatol 2004;31(10):1896–902.
6. Hjollund NH, Andersen JH, Bech P. Assessment of fatigue in chronic disease: a bibliographic study of fatigue measurement scales. Health Qual Life Outcomes 2007;5:12 Epub February 27, 2007.
7. FACIT- Fatigue Scale. Functional assessment of chronic illness therapy website. Available at: http://www.facit.org/qview/qlist.aspx. Accessed October 7, 2008.

8. Cella D, Yount S, Sorensen M, et al. Validation of the functional assessment of chronic illness therapy fatigue scale relative to other instrumentation in patients with rheumatoid arthritis. J Rheumatol 2005;32(5):811–9.

9. Dobkin BH. Fatigue versus activity-dependent fatigability in patients with central or peripheral motor impairments. Neurorehabil Neural Repair 2008;22(2):105–10.

10. Pollard LC, Choy EH, Gonzalez J, et al. Fatigue in rheumatoid arthritis reflects pain, not disease activity. Rheumatology 2006;45:885–9.

11. Guymer EK, Clauw DJ. Treatment of fatigue in fibromyalgia. Rheum Dis Clin North Am 2002;28(2):367–78.

12. Abeles AM, Pillinger MH, Solitar BM, et al. Narrative review: the pathophysiology of fibromyalgia. Ann Intern Med 2007;146(10):726–34.

13. Mease P. Fibromyalgia syndrome: review of clinical presentation, pathogenesis, outcome measures, and treatment. J Rheumatol Suppl 2005;75:6–21.

14. Geenen R, Jacobs JW. Fibromyalgia: diagnosis, pathogenesis, and treatment. Curr Opin Anaesthesiol 2001;14(5):533–9.

15. El Maghraoui A, Tellal S, Achemlal L, et al. Bone turnover and hormonal perturbations in patients with fibromyalgia. Clin Exp Rheumatol 2006;24(4):428–31.

16. Buskila D, Press J. Neuroendocrine mechanisms in fibromyalgia-chronic fatigue. Best Pract Res Clin Rheumatol 2001;15(5):747–58.

17. Ozgocmen S, Ozyurt H, Sogut S, et al. Current concepts in the pathophysiology of fibromyalgia: the potential role of oxidative stress and nitric oxide. Rheumatol Int 2006;26(7):585–97.

18. Zautra AJ, Fasman R, Parish BP, et al. Daily fatigue in women with osteoarthritis, rheumatoid arthritis,and fibromyalgia. Pain 2007;128:128–35.

19. Hamilton NA, Affleck G, Tennen H, et al. Fibromyalgia: the role of sleep in affect and in negative event reactivity and recovery. Health Psychol 2008;27(4):490–7.

20. Klippel JH, Weyand CM, Wortmann RL. Primer on the rheumatic diseases. 11th edition. Atlanta (GA): Arthritis Foundation; 1997. p. 191.

21. Moldofsky H. The significance, assessment, and management of nonrestorative sleep in fibromyalgia syndrome. CNS Spectr 2008;13(3 Suppl 5):22–6.

22. Moldofsky H. The significance of the sleeping-waking brain for the understanding of widespread musculoskeletal pain and fatigue in fibromyalgia syndrome and allied syndromes. Joint Bone Spine 2008;75(4):397–402.

23. Katz RS, Heard AR, Mills M, et al. The prevalence and clinical impact of reported cognitive difficulties (Fibrofog) in patients with rheumatic disease with and without fibromyalgia. J Clin Rheumatol 2004;10(2):53–8.

24. Leavitt F, Katz RS, Mills M, et al. Cognitive and dissociative manifestations in fibromyalgia. J Clin Rheumatol 2002;8(2):77–84.

25. Glass JM. Fibromyalgia and cognition. J Clin Psychiatry 2008;69(Suppl 2):20–4.

26. Nishishinya B, Urrútia G, Walitt B, et al. Amitriptyline in the treatment of fibromyalgia: a systematic review of its efficacy. Rheumatology (Oxford) 2008;47(12): 1741–6.

27. Tofferi JK, Jackson JL, O'Malley PG. Treatment of fibromyalgia with cyclobenzaprine: A meta-analysis. Arthritis Rheum 2004;51(1):9–13.

28. Arnold LM, Russell IJ, Diri EW, et al. A 14-week, randomized, double-blinded, placebo-controlled monotherapy trial of pregabalin in patients with fibromyalgia. J Pain 2008;9(9):792–805.

29. Mease PJ, Russell IJ, Arnold LM, et al. A randomized, double-blind, placebo-controlled, phase III trial of pregabalin in the treatment of patients with fibromyalgia. J Rheumatol 2008;35(3):502–14.

30. Russell IJ, Mease PJ, Smith TR, et al. Efficacy and safety of duloxetine for treatment of fibromyalgia in patients with or without major depressive disorder: results from a 6-month, randomized, double-blind, placebo-controlled, fixed-dose trial. Pain 2008;136(3):432–44.

31. Ottonello M. Cognitive-behavioral interventions in rheumatic diseases. G Ital Med Lav Ergon 2007;29(1 Suppl A):A19–23.

32. García J, Simón MA, Durán M, et al. Differential efficacy of a cognitive-behavioral intervention versus pharmacological treatment in the management of fibromyalgic syndrome. Psychol Health Med 2006;11(4):498–506.

33. Starlanyl D, Copeland ME. Fibromyalgia & chronic myofascial pain: a survival manual. 2nd edition. Oakland (CA): New Harbinger Publications; 2001. p. 119–27.

34. Lowry TJ, Pakenham KI. Health-related quality of life in chronic fatigue syndrome: predictors of physical functioning and psychological distress. Psychol Health Med 2008;13(2):222–38.

35. Gur A, Oktayoglu P. Central nervous system abnormalities in fibromyalgia and chronic fatigue syndrome: new concepts in treatment. Curr Pharm Des 2008; 14(13):1274–94.

36. Fukuda. The chronic fatigue syndrome: a comprehensive approach to its definition and study. Ann Intern Med 1994;121:953–9.

37. Double blind trial of duloxetine in chronic fatigue syndrome, 2008. Clinical Trials gov. Available at: http://www.clinicaltrials.gov/ct2/show/NCT00375973%3Fterm%3Dduloxetine%2C%2Bchronic%2Bfatigue%2Bsyndrome&rank%3D1.   Updated September 23, 2008. Accessed September 24, 2008.

38. Kumar R. Approved and investigational uses of modafinil: an evidence-based review. Drugs 2008;68(13):1803–39.

39. Price JR, Mitchell E, Tidy E, et al. Cognitive behaviour therapy for chronic fatigue syndrome in adults. Cochrane Database Syst Rev 2008;16(3):CD001027.

40. Nijs J, Thielemans A. Kinesiophobia and symptomatology in chronic fatigue syndrome: a psychometric study of two questionnaires. Psychol Psychother 2008;81(Pt 3):273–83.

41. Huyser BA, Parker JC, Thoreson R, et al. Predictors of subjective fatigue among individuals with rheumatoid arthritis. Arthritis Rheum 1998;41(12):2230–7.

42. Wolfe F, Michaud K, Pincus T. Fatigue, rheumatoid arthritis, and anti-tumor necrosis factor therapy: an investigation in 24,831 patients. J Rheumatol 2004; 31(11):2115–20.

43. Weinblatt ME, Keystone EC, Furst DE, et al. Adalimumab, a fully human anti–tumor necrosis factor monoclonal antibody, for the treatment of rheumatoid arthritis in patients taking concomitant methotrexate—the ARMADA trial. Arthritis Rheum 2006;54(9):2793–806.

44. Cohen SB, Emery P, Greenwald MW 2nd, et al. Rituximab for rheumatoid arthritis refractory to anti–tumor necrosis factor therapy. Arthritis rheum 2006;54(9): 2793–806.

45. Keystone E, Burmester GR, Furie R, et al. Improvement in patient-reported outcomes in a rituximab trial in patients with severe rheumatoid arthritis refractory to anti–tumor necrosis factor therapy. Arthritis Rheum 2008;59(6):785–93.

46. Mease PJ, Revicki DA, Szechinski J, et al. Improved health-related quality of life for patients with active rheumatoid arthritis receiving rituximab—results of the dose-ranging assessment: international clinical evaluation of rituximab in rheumatoid arthritis (DANCER) trial. J Rheumatol 2008;35(1):20–30.

47. Davis MC, Zautra AJ, Younger J, et al. Chronic stress and regulation of cellular markers of inflammation in rheumatoid arthritis: implications for fatigue. Brain Behav Immun 2008;22(1):24–32.
48. Murphy SL, Smith DM, Clauw DJ, et al. The impact of momentary pain and fatigue on physical activity in women with osteoarthritis. Arthritis Rheum 2008;59(6): 849–56.
49. Sale JE, Gignac M, Hawker G. The relationship between disease symptoms, life events, coping and treatment, and depression among older adults with osteoarthritis. J Rheumatol 2008;35(2):335–42.
50. Gignac MA, Davis AM, Hawker G, et al. "What do you expect? You're just getting older": a comparison of perceived osteoarthritis-related and aging-related health experiences in middle- and older-age adults. Arthritis Rheum 2006;55(6):905–12.
51. Power JD, Badley EM, French MR, et al. Fatigue in osteoarthritis: a qualitative study. BMC Musculoskelet Disord 2008;9:63.
52. Brosseau L, Wells GA, Tugwell P, et al. Ottawa Panel evidence-based clinical practice guidelines for aerobic fitness exercises in the management of fibromyalgia: part 1. Phys Ther 2008;88(7):857–71.
53. Brosseau L, Wells GA, Tugwell P, et al. Ottawa Panel evidence-based clinical practice guidelines for strengthening exercises in the management of fibromyalgia: part 2. Phys Ther 2008;88(7):873–86.
54. Valkeinen H, Alén M, Häkkinen A, et al. Effects of concurrent strength and endurance training on physical fitness and symptoms in postmenopausal women with fibromyalgia: a randomized controlled trial. Arch Phys Med Rehabil 2008;89(9): 1660–6.
55. Ottawa Panel. Ottawa panel evidence-based clinical practice guidelines for therapeutic exercises and manual therapy in the management of osteoarthritis. Phys Ther 2005;85(9):907–71.
56. Ottawa Panel. Ottawa Panel evidence-based clinical practice guidelines for therapeutic exercises in the management of rheumatoid arthritis in adults. Phys Ther 2004;84(10):934–72.
57. Neuberger GB, Aaronson LS, Gajewski B, et al. Predictors of exercise and effects of exercise on symptoms, function, aerobic fitness, and disease outcomes of rheumatoid arthritis. Arthritis Rheum 2007;57(6):943–52.
58. de Jong Z, Munneke M, Zwinderman AH, et al. Long term high intensity exercise and damage of small joints in rheumatoid arthritis. Ann Rheum Dis 2004;63(11): 1399–405.
59. van den Ende CH, Breedveld FC, le Cessie S, et al. Effect of intensive exercise on patients with active rheumatoid arthritis: a randomised clinical trial. Ann Rheum Dis 2000;59(8):615–21.
60. van den Ende CH, Hazes JM, le Cessie S, et al. Comparison of high and low intensity training in well controlled rheumatoid arthritis. Results of a randomised clinical trial. Ann Rheum Dis 1996;55(11):798–805.
61. Bilberg A, Ahlmén M, Mannerkorpi K. Moderately intensive exercise in a temperate pool for patients with rheumatoid arthritis: a randomized controlled study. Rheumatology (Oxford) 2005;44(4):502–8.
62. Pollo FE, Jackson RW. Knee bracing for unicompartmental osteoarthritis. J Am Acad Orthop Surg 2006;14(1):5–11.
63. Warden SJ, Hinman RS, Watson MA Jr, et al. Patellar taping and bracing for the treatment of chronic knee pain: a systematic review and meta-analysis. Arthritis Rheum 2008;59(1):73–83.

64. Hammond A, Freeman K. One-year outcomes of a randomized controlled trial of an educational-behavioural joint protection programme for people with rheumatoid arthritis. Rheumatology (Oxford) 2001;40(9):1044–51.
65. Barry MA, Purser J, Hazleman R, et al. Effect of energy conservation and joint protection education in rheumatoid arthritis. Br J Rheumatol 1994;33(12): 1171–4.
66. Wolfe F, Smythe HA, Yunus MB. The American College of Rheumatology 1990 criteria for the classification of fibromyalgia. Repot of the multicenter criteria committee. Arthritis Rheum 1990;33:160–72.

Fatigue in Cardiopulmonary Disease

Matthew N. Bartels, MD, MPH

KEYWORDS

• Fatigue • Cardiac rehabilitation • Pulmonary rehabilitation
• Exercise • Cardiac disease • Pulmonary disease

A very prominent symptom in most cardiac and pulmonary conditions is fatigue. It is present in up to 69% to 82% of patients with cardiac disease and up to 68% to 80% of patients with pulmonary disease.[1–4] This is second only to breathlessness in patients with both cardiac and pulmonary conditions. Whenever a patient with either of these conditions presents, a clinician should not only look to treat the underlying disease but also assess fatigue and seek to ameliorate the symptoms. Of great concern in cardiac and pulmonary disease is the issue of the role of central versus peripheral causes of fatigue. Clearly, the hypoperfusion, altered metabolism, hypoxemia, and hypercapnia seen in cardiopulmonary disease are obvious causes of peripheral fatigue, but the issue of central causes, although somewhat controversial, may need to be addressed as well. Depression, anxiety, and fear all play a role in the fatigue seen in patients with cardiopulmonary disease and need to be considered in treatment plans. The full discussion of the role of these central causes of fatigue is beyond the scope of this review, but it should be kept in mind whenever caring for patients with cardiopulmonary disease who have symptoms of fatigue.

The major direct causes of fatigue in cardiac and pulmonary patients fall into 3 areas, 2 of which are addressed closely in this review. The role of primary cardiac and pulmonary dysfunction as a cause of fatigue is critical to understand, as these conditions may be present in patients with other major conditions, such as stroke or peripheral vascular disease, and may further contribute to those disabilities. The role of medications is also important, especially in cardiac patients, as medications to prevent or reduce cardiac events often have side effects that cause fatigue. It is important for the clinician to be aware of these side effects and to instruct his or her patients about them. The third area, central causes of fatigue, also play an important role, but are not discussed here. Treatment modifications and exercise often help to ameliorate the limitations created by the fatigue and increase the patient's capacity

Supported by the Vidda Foundation.
Department of Rehabilitation Medicine, Columbia College of Physicians and Surgeons, Unit #38, 630 West 168th Street, Columbia University, New York, NY 10032, USA
E-mail address: mnb4@columbia.edu

Phys Med Rehabil Clin N Am 20 (2009) 389–404
doi:10.1016/j.pmr.2008.12.002
1047-9651/08/$ – see front matter © 2009 Elsevier Inc. All rights reserved.

to perform exercise with less functional limitations in the face of his or her disease and treatment limitations.

ASSESSMENT FOR FATIGUE IN THE CARDIOPULMONARY PATIENT

When a patient with cardiac or pulmonary disease presents, a common primary presenting complaint is fatigue. If a patient has dyspnea with exertion, he or she will also often disclose having a secondary symptom of fatigue if the clinician asks. These symptoms may actually be similar to depression, with a decrease in interest in usual activity, a feeling of exhaustion all the time, and a marked decline in overall activity. The decreased activity then accelerates the process of fatigue, and the patient progresses to immobility. The questions that a clinician needs to ask are rather straightforward during the examination.

1. Do you feel tired most of the time or all of the time?
2. Have you decreased participation in leisure activities or occupational activities due to exhaustion?
3. Have you had a decline in the level of activity that you do on a daily basis over the last 6 months?
4. Are there activities that you cannot perform at this time that you used to be able to do 6 months to a year ago, or before you fell ill, that you do not do now due to tiredness or exhaustion?
5. Do you go to bed earlier every day than you used to 6 months to a year ago or before you became ill?

If a patient answers yes to more than 1 of these questions, he or she is likely experiencing symptoms of fatigue.

Fatigue in Cardiac Disease

One of the most common causes of fatigue in cardiac disease is seen in association with myocardial infarction (MI). An unusual feature of the presentation of fatigue after acute MI is that it is much more common in women than in men. In a study of acute coronary syndromes, fatigue was a presenting complaint in 18% of women and 9% of men.[5] The post-infarct fatigue syndrome was also associated with more severe fatigue when present in women compared with that in men. The causes of this gender difference are not clear.[6] Still, it is important to recognize that fatigue and "tiredness" are atypical symptoms that are more common in women who are having an acute myocardial event, and if unexplained by other causes, they should make the practitioner consider evaluation for cardiac disease in individuals at risk.[7] Possible speculation on mechanisms includes depression and anxiety and effects of hormonal changes, but these have not yet been elucidated.

Chronically, after an acute myocardial event, fatigue is even more commonly seen than that during the acute onset of infarction. The hypothesized causes of this increase in fatigue are multifactorial and are still unknown in many cases. Likewise, fatigue is also more common in individuals with congestive heart failure (CHF) and is often a primary feature of the condition. Interestingly, the symptom of fatigue is often present even without overt cardiac dysfunction or evidence of either systolic or diastolic dysfunction in both patients with post-MI syndromes and in patients with CHF. This has led investigators to try to elucidate the possible causes of CHF-related fatigue but with little clear success. Since the symptoms of fatigue are often vague and can overlap with any other aspects of advanced cardiac disease, there is often a great deal of difficulty in distinguishing between physiologic effects of decreased cardiac output, deconditioning, aging, and underlying mood disorders in specific cases.[8] Highlighting the central role of fatigue in CHF, several studies have defined CHF syndromes based on inclusion of at least 2 of the following: dyspnea, *fatigue,* orthopnea, paroxysmal nocturnal dyspnea, third heart sound, jugular venous distention, rales, and leg edema. The biological mechanisms of fatigue that may be a part of heart failure include the following possible areas.

A large component of fatigue in cardiac disease can come from depression, which is commonly seen in both CHF and after MI. As a correlation of psychological state and fatigue, for any patient with cardiac disease, the presence of depression greatly increases the likelihood of fatigue.[9–11] Additionally, the presence of depression increases mortality among all cardiac patients. It has been hypothesized that the mechanism for fatigue in depression and in cardiac disease may actually share several mechanisms. Some of the commonly shared abnormalities between patients with fatigue in cardiac disease (without depression) and patients with pure depression (without cardiac disease) include sympathoadrenal dysregulation, decreased heart rate variability, platelet dysfunction, and negative health behaviors. In addition to these changes, there also may be an attenuation of baroreflex control of heart rate and a contribution from immune system dysfunction.[12] Attenuation of the baroreceptor reflex and loss of heart rate variability are associated with premature death in patients with cardiac disease, highlighting the importance of treatment of the fatigue if at all possible, since this may be a treatable risk factor in cardiac disease. These studies also correlated the autonomic dysfunction seen in the depressed population with an increase in cardiovascular mortality, further strengthening the importance of efforts to improve the autonomic function.

Additionally, hypothalamic-pituitary-adrenal (HPA) axis abnormalities in purely cardiac and purely depressed patients can share similarities in the alterations seen in stress responses. To have a normal stress response, there needs to be a synthesis of corticotropin-releasing hormone (CRH) in the hypothalamus, which then causes an increase in adrenocorticotropic (ACTH) hormone via the hypothalamo-hypophyseal portal system. The ACTH in turn causes an increase in secretion of catecholamines and cortisol from the adrenal glands, which then regulate the HPA axis via a feedback mechanism. Depression and cardiac disease both cause an excess of cortisol secretion and alterations in CRH and ACTH concentrations—in a pattern that mimics stress. This leads to an excess of sympathetic tone, which in turn leads to a reflex increase in heart rate in the "stress mode," consistent with levels that are observed in untreated CHF and post-MI patients. In tandem with these findings is a decrease in heart rate variability in both depressed patients and in individuals with cardiac disease, which is known to be associated with increased risk of sudden death after MI.[13–16] Similar findings of alteration in baroreflex responses are also present in patients with cardiac disease and depression, most of whom also have symptoms of fatigue.[17]

Immune system dysfunction is also seen to have a role in fatigue in patients with cardiac disease. There is a role of alteration in cytokines and in the regulation of immune function that happens in both depression and with cardiac disease. Specifically, there is an association of excess of tumor necrosis factor alpha (TNF-α)[18] and interleukin 1-beta[19] (IL-1-β) and the symptoms of fatigue. A similar pattern of increased cytokines is also seen in patients after coronary surgery, after MI, and with heart failure. This alteration of cytokines and increased TNF-α may play a role in post-surgical or post-MI fatigue, which is seen in a great number of patients.[20,21] The final mechanism that the immune dysregulation may have on the control of fatigue in cardiac patients may be through the effects that dysregulation of immune function can have on the HPA axis with alteration of catecholamines and subsequent increased circulating cortisol. It has been hypothesized that myocardial disease, specifically infarction, can lead to immune activation with the cascade or increased TNF-α and IL-1-β, leading to deregulation of the prefrontal cortex and producing limbic dysfunction with subsequent mood changes (depression) and direct increase in the humoral factors, which can lead to increased fatigue.[22,23] A side effect of this is also an increase in cardiac events, including arrhythmias and increased MI. Reversal of the fatigue has not been clearly shown to improve the cardiac events but has been associated with an improvement in the humoral markers discussed previously.

Another consideration in the relationship of fatigue and cardiac disease is the role that fatigue has as a risk factor for further cardiac events. In the Copenhagen Heart study, vital exhaustion—a marker of fatigue with associated depressive symptoms—was found to be an independent risk factor for ischemic heart disease.[24] Patients with depression were nearly twice as likely to develop subsequent cardiac events and had an increased overall mortality even for noncardiac events. The increased incidence of events and death was thought to be possibly mediated by the mechanisms mentioned already, including autonomic dysfunction, immune dysregulation, and altered platelet function. The same increase in events was found for patients who underwent percutaneous transluminal coronary angioplasty with an increased incidence in new cardiac events in patients who reported vital exhaustion.[25]

Fatigue in Pulmonary Disease

Just as in patients with cardiac disease, patients with chronic obstructive pulmonary disease (COPD), interstitial lung disease (ILD), and other lung conditions often present with fatigue as a prominent symptom. In patients with COPD, fatigue is second only to breathlessness in incidence as a major symptom, being present in 68% to 80% of patients.[2,4] Fatigue is also commonly seen in ILD, and assessment for the presence of fatigue is an integral part of the assessment of quality of life in lung disease.[26,27] Although the exact cause of fatigue in these patients with chronic lung disease is not clearly understood, there are some aspects that overlap with other chronic diseases and some that are unique to lung disease.

The features of fatigue with COPD and ILD that are shared with other chronic diseases include muscle weakness, early fatigue (exhaustion with exercise), muscle wasting, and decreased muscle function. This is seen in the same way as in cardiac disease. There are thought to be several contributing factors to this constellation of fatigue symptoms, including semistarvation (both cardiac and pulmonary cachexia), reduced physical activity, and aging, along with the effects of lung failure. Additionally, patients with chronic lung disease often exist in a chronic catabolic state and have muscle changes that can resemble those seen in patients with anorexia and starvation.[28] Another factor that can further increase this catabolic state is the effects of medications and the effects of immobility imposed by frequent hospitalizations and the limitations on activity from the lung disease itself. Patients with lung disease will often enter a spiral of decreasing weight after a series of hospitalizations with intubations and periods of decreased nutrition, high-dose steroids, and courses of broad-spectrum antibiotics.

Another cause of the fatigue that is so often present in COPD may be related to dyspnea and the effort of breathing. Patients with severe COPD may have no relief from the effort of breathing and develop anxiety and depression, which compound their fatigue.[29] The mechanism of a large component of respiratory fatigue is related to the effort of breathing itself. The work of breathing is increased in COPD, because all aspects of the ventilatory cycle are active, since exhalation no longer is a passive activity due to air trapping. This increase in the work of breathing can increase resting metabolic demand up to twice the normal level.[29] To further complicate this fatigue from increased work, there is a chronic increase in metabolic demand, which, coupled with the altered nutrition seen in patients with severe COPD, can lead to muscle wasting and malnourishment discussed previously. This leads to muscular weakness and increased perception of work, and a deadly downward spiral can ensue.

In addition to the increased metabolic demand, there are also limitations with appetite and changes in the ability to maintain lean body mass. The limitations to maintaining adequate dietary intake are multifactorial. Mechanical difficulty with eating comes from a combination of pressure on the diaphragm from a large meal, decreasing ventilatory reserve, and the increased metabolic demand of digestion, causing the patient to have more dyspnea.[29] Decreased appetite from medications and the effects of glucocorticoids increasing fat percentage with a loss of lean body mass also contribute. The result is a pulmonary cachexia, which cycles with progressively more lean body mass loss into a chronic and potentially lethal spiral. This progressive cachexia and loss of lean body mass also lead to weakness of the muscles of respiration (diaphragm and accessory muscles of ventilation, which are extensively used for patients with COPD), leading to a loss of ventilatory capacity, which in turn leads to increased symptoms of dyspnea and chronic fatigue.[30] Finally, it is hypothesized that there may also be biochemical pathways contributing to this chronic weight loss, but these are not clearly understood at this point.

Another factor in the development of fatigue in COPD is the possible presence of obstructive sleep apnea (OSA) along with lung disease.[31,32] This is a relatively common concurrence of conditions, and one of the most prominent effects of sleep deprivation from OSA is an increase in fatigue, above and beyond the effects of COPD itself. The most effective intervention for a patient who presents with both conditions is to treat both COPD and OSA simultaneously and aggressively. Nocturnal, noninvasive, bilevel ventilation is a hallmark of this treatment and will help with OSA directly and may provide nocturnal rest for the ventilatory muscles fatigued by the increased effort of ventilation with obstructive lung disease. As evidence of the relationship of the conditions, when appropriately treated, most patients experience a marked improvement in fatigue. An additional interesting finding in individuals with both OSA and COPD is that fatigue is increased in direct proportion to decreased activity and fatigue is not directly related to the severity of OSA.[31,32]

There is also an elevated incidence of depression in patients with OSA and COPD. This depression may be difficult to tease out from the physiologic effects of apnea.[33] Another common factor with both OSA and COPD is the effects of hypercarbia and hypoxemia on the individual, with both abnormalities causing fatigue.

For patients with ILD, the mechanism of fatigue may be due to depression, muscle wasting, medications, and associated collagen, vascular, or autoimmune diseases, along with the effects of immobility. Medications that are most often associated with fatigue include corticosteroids and chemotherapeutic agents, such as azathioprine (Imuran), cyclophosphamide (Cytoxan), and interferon. Just as in COPD, added to these effects is the extra effort of breathing, possible presence of hypoxemia, and the development of pulmonary hypertension with subsequent right heart failure. The constellation of problems can all be seen in a single patient as the disease progresses, and, in part, this is why aggressive treatment with oxygen may help. However, no matter what treatments are offered, the onset of fatigue is likely. Just as in COPD, the extra work of breathing, combined with weakened musculature, can contribute to the onset of fatigue. Unlike in COPD, the increased work of breathing in ILD is not due to the loss of elasticity and subsequent active exhalation but rather due to the loss of compliance of the lungs. As the disease progresses, the lungs become very stiff and excessive force is needed to ventilate them, leading to smaller tidal volumes with increased inefficiency of breathing.

The effects of autoimmune conditions and collagen vascular diseases on fatigue are due to many mechanisms similar to those discussed in cardiac disease with increased cytokines and subsequent dysregulation of the immune system. High doses of glucocorticoid medications are also often used to treat concomitant collagen vascular disease, and these medications also have a role in causing fatigue. The underlying autoimmune disease can also directly damage muscles, causing direct muscle weakness and associated fatigue.[34] An example of this is connective tissue disease-associated pulmonary fibrosis, which is seen in up to 89% of patients with mixed connective tissue disease, whereas up to 69% of patients have pulmonary function test abnormalities.[34] The histopathology of lung involvement is similar to usual interstitial pneumonitis or nonspecific interstitial pneumonitis in most cases. In some rarer cases, ILD may be due to the treatment for the disease, most commonly when patients receive methotrexate as a part of the treatment of their autoimmune disorder.[35]

Just as in patients with cardiac disease, patients with pulmonary disease can develop fatigue after surgery. Additionally, there is the possibility of fatigue in the setting of lung cancer and after the treatments that are instituted for cancer—surgery, chemotherapy, and radiation therapy. These treatments are all known to contribute to fatigue but will not be discussed in detail here. Other sources are available to review the serious consequences of cancer on lung function and the effects of medications, and interested readers can find the details in specific texts that relate to these disorders.[35] The usual effect is one of ILD and the associated abnormalities discussed earlier.

ROLE OF DEPRESSION AND ANXIETY

Depression, anxiety, and fear underlie all of the cardiopulmonary conditions that may lead to the presence of fatigue, and these affective disorders may actually augment the symptoms of fatigue when they are present. As stated above, not only is depression well known to be associated with fatigue but also fatigue is often one of the cardinal presenting symptoms of depression. The major point to remember with patients affected by cardiopulmonary disease is that whenever fatigue seems to be out of proportion to the degree of underlying disease, an assessment for depression or anxiety should be considered. When it is present, treatment of depression can help to alleviate the symptoms of fatigue, allowing for an increase in physical activity, which will also improve fatigue.

ROLE OF MEDICATIONS IN FATIGUE IN CARDIOPULMONARY DISEASE

Among medications for the treatment of cardiac disease, historically, beta blockers and diuretics have been thought to be associated with the highest incidence of the side effect of fatigue. Evaluations of calcium channel blockers, angiotensin-converting enzyme (ACE) inhibitors, and antiarrhythmics have sporadic reports of fatigue, but the beta blockers are most often reported to be associated with fatigue.

Interestingly, recent re-evaluation of the side effects of beta blockers has come to dispute the "commonly known" association of beta blockade and fatigue. Several recent studies have shown that the physiologic benefits of the beta blockers actually decreased fatigue in patients with coronary artery disease (CAD) and heart failure when used appropriately.[36,37] Similarly, patients using diuretics that maintained euvolemia and normal electrolyte balance did not experience increased fatigue. This means that physicians treating patients with cardiac disease who are found to have fatigue should not automatically attribute the symptoms of fatigue to the medications. Instead, improved treatment of their underlying condition or evaluation for depression or another cause of increased fatigue should be considered.

Pulmonary medications do not usually have an association with fatigue, with the exception of glucocorticoids. The effects of steroids on fatigue can be usually attributed to the effects on muscle catabolism, weight gain, and the changes on affect, particularly the onset of depression. Patients with high-dose steroid treatment are most likely to have these adverse effects, so minimizing the dosage is important. Similarly, patients with transplantation are also likely to be on high doses of prednisone and have these associated symptoms.

The effects of medications on fatigue are of particular interest in both pulmonary and cardiac transplant patients. A common symptom in this population of patients after transplantation is that they have continued fatigue long after their transplant and recovery, even with good graft function. This fatigue is never as severe as before their transplant, but the energy level and exercise capacity remain reduced.[38] In cardiac transplant patients, there is a decreased cardiac output due to denervation of the heart with resultant cardiac dysfunction that leads to a lower maximum cardiac output, with coincident reduction in exercise capacity.[40] Pulmonary transplant patients do not have cardiac limitation but have decreased exercise capacity.[35] In a large part, the transplant medications themselves contribute to the decreased capacity (ie, the effect of glucocorticoids from decreased muscle strength and muscle mass).

Another key contribution to decreased exercise capacity is the effect of calcineurin inhibitor (CI) medications. Practically all transplant patients are treated with a regimen that includes both glucocorticoids and CI. The most commonly used CIs are cyclosporine and tacrolimus. Although there are some differences, all of the CIs inhibit the function of calcineurin, which plays an important role in the regeneration of muscle, and the CIs thus inhibit the formation of type I muscle fibers.[39–41] Cyclosporin has also been associated with mitochondrial dysfunction and the developments of myopathy. The mechanisms appear to involve inhibition of mitochondrial respiration, and impairment of the enzyme function of succinate dehydrogenase has been found.[42,43] The fatigue may well be related to this effect on mitochondrial function and may explain the high prevalence of fatigue in these patients. Unfortunately, for the treatment of fatigue, reduction of the medications is not an option for these patients. The best compromise is to treat them symptomatically with exercise and encourage maintenance of lean body mass, while coordinating with the transplant service to try to minimize the immunosuppressive medications as much as possible. Fortunately, the levels of medications often decrease markedly in the first year after transplantation if there is no rejection, only to be boosted in times of possible rejection.

A summary of the potential effects of some commonly used cardiac and pulmonary medication classes is seen in **Table 1**.

Possible Therapeutic Interventions

Patients with cardiac and pulmonary disease commonly have fatigue for the reasons discussed earlier, some of which are directly due to their disease, some of which are due to metabolic and other effects of their condition, and some of which may be due to complications in the treatment of their disease. Fortunately, some of the causes of fatigue can be ameliorated through treatment. In the management of affective causes of fatigue, it is essential to treat depression, anxiety, and fear if they exist in all cardiopulmonary patients. This alone may help increase the patient's energy level to help facilitate involvement with other treatments such as exercise that will further improve the patient's fatigue. For depression and anxiety, treatment should include both

Table 1
Common medications used to treat cardiac and pulmonary disease that may cause fatigue

Cardiac Disease	Mechanism for Fatigue	Effect on Fatigue
Beta blocker	Decreased sympathetic activation	No clear evidence in recent studies
ACE inhibitors	Unclear mechanism	Sporadic reports
Diuretics	Metabolic disarray Dehydration	No effect as long as electrolytes and fluid balance normal
Antihypertensives	Lowered blood pressure Decreased ability to mount a sympathetic response	Direct effect of low blood pressure
Pulmonary disease		
Glucocorticoids	Muscle weakness Hyperglycemia Hypertension Weight gain Mood changes	Can clearly increase fatigue through a combination of physiologic effects
Interferon	Fever Malaise	May cause fatigue directly
Cytotoxic agents	Anemia Malaise Exhaustion	May cause fatigue directly
Post-transplant		
Glucocorticoids	Muscle weakness Hyperglycemia Hypertension Weight gain Mood changes	Can clearly increase fatigue
Calcineurin inhibitors	Decreased muscle contractility Decreased type 1 fiber generation Impaired function of succinate dehydrogenase	Associated with muscle weakness and fatigue
Cytotoxic agents	Anemia Malaise Exhaustion	May cause fatigue directly
Antihypertensive agents	Needed to counteract elevation of blood pressure from glucocorticoids and calcineurin inhibitors Lowered blood pressure	Direct effect of low blood pressure

pharmacologic therapy as well as psychotherapy. The issue is to try to relieve psychomotor retardation and the central effects of depression that cause fatigue. The full discussion of the effect of depression on fatigue and how to treat it is covered in other sources.

The treatment of muscle weakness and muscle fiber fatigue is possible and can assist in the relief of fatigue in cardiopulmonary disease. The muscle dysfunction that exists with lung disease responds to both the treatment of the underlying condition as well as to exercise to directly strengthen muscle and increase muscle fiber endurance. As an example, in COPD, leg fatigue is a prominent symptom and is seen in up to one-third of patients. Associated with the leg fatigue there is also a decrease of up to 20% in muscle twitch force.[44,45] This loss of strength and endurance leads to an increase in symptoms of fatigue, as every activity is nearer the maximum strength of the individual. Treating bronchospasm and dyspnea alone does not resolve the issues of fatigue, and it is only with a combination of exercise that there is even more significant improvement.[46,47] For patients with COPD, treatment of the underlying COPD with lung volume reduction surgery (LVRS) can lead to an improvement in function but has no clear effect on the underlying symptoms of fatigue.[48] Exercise capacity with LVRS increased 10% to 15%, and pulmonary function testing showed improved forced expiratory volume in 1 second (from 59 to 71% predicted), but the perceived measures of fatigue with exertion were unchanged. However, this same population of patients experience a significant improvement in ratings of perceived fatigue with exertion when they exercise,[49] and they also had associated levels of improvements in exercise capacity without any improvements in pulmonary function. Similar findings exist for exercise with ILD.

The method of exercise for patients with pulmonary limitation should emphasize endurance training. The level of dyspnea that patients experience is such that they may not continue to exercise if the level of exertion is too high, and it is consistency in exercise with a dedication to increased endurance that yields the best benefits.[48,49] Additionally, the use of supplemental oxygen is essential to limit fatigue, both with exercise training and with activity. Chronic hypoxemia will lead to fatigue on its own, and the avoidance of this additional factor in fatigue is essential in the management of both dyspnea and the prevention of chronic hypoxemia with its associated fatigue.

For patients with cardiac disease, similar findings exist, and treatment of the underlying cardiac condition is important, as it will allow for better perfusion and improved function with decreased fatigue. This is especially true in ischemic disease and in CHF.

TREATMENT OF OBESITY

Finally, although it has not yet been mentioned, treatment of obesity, if present, is essential in helping to manage fatigue in cardiopulmonary patients. Deconditioning and excess weight are epidemic in our society and are the root cause of a great deal of fatigue, even without other underlying conditions. Cardiopulmonary patients are not immune to developing deconditioning and obesity. In fact, these groups of patients may actually have a higher degree of both due to inactivity from their cardiopulmonary limitations. With pulmonary disease, dyspnea is the usual limiting factor, and with cardiac disease, both dyspnea and chest pain will limit activity. Therefore, any program of therapy that is aimed to reduce fatigue in cardiopulmonary patients needs to address weight reduction to increase the likelihood of success.

The treatment approaches for weight reduction are outside of the scope of this review, but most of the common approaches used for healthy individuals will also work for patients with cardiopulmonary disease. Practitioners are urged to be familiar with local resources so that they can avail themselves of assistance in helping to manage weight loss.

PRINCIPLES OF EXERCISE FOR PATIENTS WITH FATIGUE IN CHRONIC CARDIAC AND PULMONARY DISEASE

A properly designed cardiac or pulmonary program will start with an assessment of the primary condition. For patients with cardiac disease, an evaluation of cardiac function and limitations is essential for safety and to maximize the effectiveness of the cardiac rehabilitation program. Control of CHF and ischemia is required, and the patient should have an assessment of maximal exercise capacity to help with safety assessment and planning for the appropriate level of sustainable exercise. For pulmonary patients, the patient should be on an optimized regimen of bronchodilation and should be on an appropriate level of supplemental oxygen. It is also important to limit the amounts of systemic steroids as much as possible. When present, the patient's anxiety should also be controlled, because this can contribute to a limitation for exercise. Treatment of anxiety can include pharmaceutical measures, but a good rehabilitation program will also include stress management and education.[38,46,47] Guidelines for supplemental oxygen and hemodynamic parameters for the lung patients can also be directed with physiologic testing and pulmonary function testing.

Once the parameters for safe exercise are determined, patients are best placed in a supervised program initially to facilitate participation and to increase the maximal exercise that they can perform. There are several other issues that will affect the ability of the patients to participate in the exercise program.

For patients with cardiopulmonary disease, accessibility is important. This includes maintaining cost at a reasonable level and developing a continuing exercise program that is home based. Often there may need to be negotiation with insurers to assure coverage. For cardiac diseases, in situations where accessibility or insurance coverage may be difficult, home-based programs have proven effective in the maintenance of conditioning. Home-based programs also have the additional benefit of associated improvements in fatigue that are often better with home-based exercise than center-based exercise.[50] Placing exercise in community-based settings is also helpful and can be done at senior centers, community centers, schools, and residential facilities. Educational and motivational programs can also be included to maintain enthusiasm, and the socialization that occurs in the community-based settings may also help patients to overcome anxiety and depression, which contribute to their fatigue.[30]

Safety and effectiveness of the exercise program need to be assured through appropriate assessment and prescription of precautions. As discussed here, use of supplemental oxygen and appropriate monitoring for cardiac patients will help to reassure patients and allow them to exercise to an appropriate level. The effectiveness of the exercise program will also be maximized when an appropriate level of intensity and duration are achieved. Increased-duration exercise sessions that are more frequent are associated with more benefits. Additionally, exercise that is done with weight bearing and near the anaerobic threshold is more effective. A rough rule of thumb for intensity is to try to achieve sustained exercise for 30 minutes at an intensity of approximately 60% of peak performance 3 to 5 times a week.[51–53] Since upper-extremity activity causes more fatigue than that with similar-intensity leg exercise, there also needs to be a focus on arm exercise to improve upper-limb strength and endurance. A properly executed gentle exercise program for the upper body can achieve similar improvements to those with the exercise programs for lower extremities.[54]

For a complete exercise program, muscle-strengthening exercise needs to be incorporated in addition to the conditioning exercises. In patients with significant muscle weakness, such as lung disease patients who have been on long-term glucocorticoids, or in post-transplant patients, there is a need to focus on proximal and large muscle groups for strengthening. This also applies to cardiopulmonary patients who may have had prolonged hospitalizations and are in need of recovery from immobility. If possible, the exercises should include free weights as opposed to circuit training, since there is a better training effect.[55,56] For convenience and variety, effective strengthening programs can also include theraband or other forms of resistance exercises.[34,55,56]

Another element in maintaining the benefits of exercise include making sure that the patient adheres to the exercise program. Physician encouragement and patient motivation are also important.[57,58] It is essential for the fatigued cardiopulmonary patient not to have an overwhelming program that may seem too difficult to achieve. Rather than presenting a very intense and threatening series of overall goals, smaller short-term goals can be helpful and build a sense of accomplishment in the patient. Additionally, the types of exercise that the patient enjoys should be emphasized, and ones that are not comfortable should be avoided as a regular part of the program. Circuit training also introduces variety and may help to prevent injury from overuse or repetitive strain. When a patient has achieved a level of capacity, repeat exercise testing to demonstrate the new level of strength and conditioning may also help and can be in the form of a 6-minute walk test or cardiopulmonary exercise test. Some techniques that can make the actual exercise program more enjoyable include finding an exercise partner (spouse or friend), incorporating the exercise into a recreational sport, and using techniques for distraction during sustained exercise, such as television, music, or conversation. Patients who are enrolled in a formal program also often find camaraderie in the exercise program and so can increase their adherence by being more excited to come for the socialization that their exercise program provides.[38,55]

Once the cardiopulmonary patients have achieved a degree of conditioning with the associated improvement in fatigue, they should be encouraged to think of incorporating exercise as a part of their ongoing overall health care plan. The physician and other members of the health care team need to be unwavering in their support for exercise, and it is important to also enlist the patient's family as a support. Educating the patient on the role of exercise in treating the underlying cardiopulmonary disease and in combating the side effects of medications is also important. A summary of the effects of exercise on fatigue in chronic cardiopulmonary disease is presented in **Table 2**.

POTENTIAL AREAS FOR RESEARCH IN CARDIOPULMONARY FATIGUE

Since there are still numerous areas that have not been defined in the role of fatigue in cardiac and pulmonary diseases, ongoing research is needed. A special consideration is that even with the recent marked improvements in treatment for cardiac and pulmonary disease, fatigue is still a major presenting symptom or part of cardiopulmonary disease. Theoretically, recent advancements in treatment have allowed for the correction of the underlying pathophysiology or even eradication of the underlying disease, thus removing the cardiac or pulmonary cause of fatigue. However, even after these interventions, the symptoms of fatigue often continue to persist for patients.

The most successful examples of definitive treatment of underlying cardiac disorders include valve replacement for valvular heart disease and revascularization for early ischemic heart disease (before MI and onset of heart failure). In these patients, there is the best chance for definitive relief of fatigue. For patients who are on medications for restoration of exercise capacity (such as intravenous inotropic agents) or supplemental oxygen, the underlying fatigue often persists. In patients who receive transplantation, there is also persistence of fatigue due to the medication regimens for prevention of resection and side effects, effectively creating an exchange of the original cardiopulmonary condition for "transplant disease." Research efforts need to be focused on attempts to improve overall function and to enhance cardiac and pulmonary function to improve fatigue symptoms, while minimizing the side effects of the treatment that cause fatigue. This combination of searching for effective

Table 2
Benefits of exercise in chronic cardiopulmonary disease

Benefits	Effect on Physiology	Subsequent Effect on Fatigue
Decreases risk of CAD mortality	Decreased cardiac events	Unclear
Decreases risk of hypertension	Lowered incidence of hypertension	Decrease
Lowers blood pressure in individuals with hypertension	Lowered blood pressure	Decrease
Maintains muscle strength	Improved muscle strength	Unclear
Maintains bone mass	Improved bone density	Unclear
Improves glycemic control	Lower blood sugar	Decrease
Improved coordination	Decreases fall risk	Unclear
Improved sense of well-being	Relieves symptoms of anxiety and depression	Decrease
Improved health-related quality of life	Improves ability to function	Unclear to decrease
Reduced risk of cancer	Less neoplasm	Unclear
Improved lipid profile	Decreased cardiovascular risk	Unclear
Increased exercise capacity	Improved ability to function	Decrease
Decreased obesity	Lowers body weight	Decrease
Improved sleep quality	Less fatigue from sleep deprivation	Decrease
Improved self-image	Lowers chance of affective disorders	Decrease

treatments for a symptom while actually using treatments that may contribute to the symptom makes the study of fatigue and its treatments very challenging.

FUTURE PROSPECTS IN FATIGUE IN CARDIOPULMONARY DISEASE

The future challenges in defining fatigue in cardiopulmonary disease are numerous. Unfortunately, as mentioned above, the research in the area of fatigue in cardiac and pulmonary disease is limited, and much still needs to be done. There is a clear role for central versus peripheral factors, and this is true of research regarding all forms of fatigue not just fatigue seen in patients with heart or lung disease. Still, the best approach for a patient with fatigue in cardiopulmonary disease is to address multiple issues simultaneously. First, there needs to be attention to maximizing the treatment of the underlying condition and minimizing the physiologic disturbances from hypoxemia, hypercarbia, and decreased cardiac output or myocardial compromise. Then there needs to be attention to contributing conditions, such as obesity, deconditioning, depression, or anxiety. Finally, there needs to be consideration of the possible effects of the treatments themselves and minimizing the possibilities that the treatments cause fatigue. Through this multifaceted approach, the clinician will best be able to help patients with their fatigue.

In conclusion, the take-home message for health care practitioners working with cardiopulmonary patients with fatigue is to have a good understanding of the underlying conditions and the possible treatment options. In addition to maximizing medical management of the cardiac and pulmonary conditions, an appropriate exercise program needs to be done, along with appropriate medication management and evaluation of and treatment for obesity, depression, anxiety, and other conditions associated with fatigue. It may not be possible to totally remove the symptom of fatigue, but with appropriate management, the symptom can be controlled sufficiently to allow patients to return to a higher level of functioning.

REFERENCES

1. Anderson H, Ward C, Eardley A, et al. The concerns of patients under palliative care and a heart failure clinic are not being met. Palliat Med 2001;15:279–86.
2. Lynn J, Teno JM, Phillips RS, et al. Perceptions by family members of the dying experience of older and seriously ill patients. Ann Intern Med 1997;126(2):97–106.
3. Nordgren L, Sorensen S. Symptoms experienced in the last six months of life in patients with end-stage heart failure. Eur J Cardiovasc Nurs 2003;2(3):213–7.
4. Skilbeck J, Mott L, Page H, et al. Palliative care in chronic obstructive airways disease: a needs assessment. Palliat Med 1998;12:245–54.
5. Milner KA, Funk M, Richards S, et al. Gender differences in symptom presentation associated with coronary heart disease. Am J Cardiol 1999;84:396–9.
6. Meshack AF, Goff DC, Chan W. Comparison of reported symptoms of acute myocardial infarction in Mexican Americans versus non-Hispanic whites (the Corpus Christi Heart Project). Am J Cardiol 1998;82:1329–32.
7. Patel H, Rosengren A, Ekman I. Symptoms in acute coronary syndromes: does sex make a difference? Am Heart J 2004;148(1):27–33.
8. Azevedo A, Bettencourt P, Pimenta J, et al. Clinical syndrome suggestive of heart failure is frequently attributable to non-cardiac disorders — population-based study. Eur J Heart Fail 2007;9:391–6.
9. Anda R, Williamson D, Jones D, et al. Depressed affect, hopelessness, and the risk of ischemic heart disease in a cohort of U.S. adults. Epidemiology 1993;4:285–94.
10. Barefoot JC, Schroll M. Symptoms of depression, acute myocardial infarction, and total mortality in a community sample. Circulation 1996;93:1976–80.
11. Everson SA, Goldberg DE, Kaplan GA, et al. Hopelessness and risk of mortality and incidence of myocardial infarction and cancer. Psychosom Med 1996;58:113–21.
12. Grippo AJ, Johnson AK. Biological mechanisms in the relationship between depression and heart disease. Neurosci Biobehav Rev 2002;26:941–62.
13. Carney RM, Saunders RD, Freedland KE, et al. Association of depression with reduced heart rate variability in coronary artery disease. Am J Cardiol 1995;76:562–4.
14. Pitzalis MV, Iacoviello M, Todarello O, et al. Depression but not anxiety influences the autonomic control of heart rate after myocardial infarction. Am Heart J 2001;141:765–71.
15. Rechlin T, Weis M, Claus D. Heart rate variability in depressed patients and differential effects of paroxetine and amitriptyline on cardiovascular autonomic function. Pharmacopsychiatry 1994;27:124–8.
16. Rechlin T, Weis M, Spitzer A, et al. Are affective disorders associated with alterations of heart rate variability? J Affect Disord 1994;32:271–5.
17. Watkins LL, Grossman P. Association of depressive symptoms with reduced baroreflex cardiac control in coronary artery disease. Am Heart J 1999;137:453–7.

18. Spriggs DR, Sherman ML, Michie H, et al. Recombinant human tumor necrosis factor administered as a 24-hour intravenous infusion. A phase 1 and pharmacology study. J Natl Cancer Inst 1988;80:1039–44.
19. Niiranen A, Laaksonen R, Iivanainen M, et al. Behavioral assessment of patients treated with alpha-interferon. Acta Psychiatr Scand 1988;78:622–6.
20. Hennein HA, Ebba H, Rodriguez JL, et al. Relationship of the proinflammatory cytokines to myocardial ischemia and dysfunction after uncomplicated coronary revascularization. J Thorac Cardiovasc Surg 1994;108:626–35.
21. Levine B, Kalman J, Mayer L, et al. Elevated circulating levels of tumor necrosis factor in severe chronic heart failure. N Engl J Med 1990;323:236–41 [Neurosci 1992;14:1–10].
22. Ter Horst GJ. TNF-alpha-induced selective cerebral endothelial leakage and increased mortality risk in postmyocardial infarction depression. Am J Physiol Heart Circ Physiol 1998;275:H1910–1.
23. Ter Horst GJ. Central autonomic control of the heart, angina, and pathogenic mechanisms of post-myocardial infarction depression. Eur J Morphol 1999;37:257–66.
24. Prescott E, Holst C, Grønbæk M, et al. Vital exhaustion as a risk factor for ischaemic heart disease and all-cause mortality in a community sample. A prospective study of 4084 men and 5479 women in the Copenhagen City Heart Study. Int J Epidemiol 2003;32:990–7.
25. Kop WJ, Appels A, Mendes de Leon CF, et al. Vital exhaustion predicts new cardiac events after successful coronary angioplasty. Psychosom Med 1994;56:281–7.
26. Swigris JJ, Kuschner WG, Jacobs SS, et al. Health-related quality of life in patients with idiopathic pulmonary fibrosis: a systematic review. Thorax 2005;60(7):588–94.
27. Trendall J, Esmond G. Fatigue in people with chronic obstructive pulmonary disease: development of an assessment tool. J Clin Nurs 2007;16:116–22.
28. Franssen FM, Wouters EF, Schols AM. The contribution of starvation, deconditioning and ageing to the observed alterations in peripheral skeletal muscle in chronic organ diseases. Clin Nutr 2002;21(1):1–14.
29. Seamark DA, Seamark CJ, Halpin DM. Palliative care in chronic obstructive pulmonary disease: a review for clinicians. J R Soc Med 2007;100(5):225–33.
30. Wouters EF. Management of severe COPD. Lancet 2004;364:883–95.
31. Hong S, Dimsdale JE. Physical activity and perception of energy and fatigue in obstructive sleep apnea. Med Sci Sports Exerc 2003;35(7):1088–92.
32. Aguillard RN, Riedel BW, Lichstein KL, et al. Daytime functioning in obstructive sleep apnea patients: exercise tolerance, subjective fatigue, and sleepiness. Appl Psychophysiol Biofeedback 1998;23:207–17.
33. Bardwell WA, Moore P, Ancoli-Israel S, et al. Fatigue in obstructive sleep apnea: driven by depressive symptoms instead of apnea severity? Am J Psychiatry 2003;160:350–5.
34. Prakash UB. Lungs in mixed connective tissue disease. J Thorac Imaging 1992;7(2):55–61.
35. Bartels MN, Mattera D. Pulmonary Complications of Cancer and its Treatment. In: Stubblefield M, O'Dell M, editors. Principles and Practices of Cancer Rehabilitation. Chapter 26. New York: Demos Medical Publishing; 2009. p. 331–48.
36. Ko DT, Hebert PR, Coffey CS, et al. Adverse effects of beta-blocker therapy for patients with heart failure: a quantitative overview of randomized trials. Arch Intern Med 2004;164:1389–94.
37. Ko DT, Hebert PR, Coffey CS, et al. Beta- blocker therapy and symptoms of depression, fatigue, and sexual dysfunction. JAMA 2002;288:351–7.

38. Bartels MN, Whiteson JH, Alba AS, et al. Cardiopulmonary rehabilitation and cancer rehabilitation. 1. Cardiac rehabilitation review. Arch Phys Med Rehabil 2006;87(3 Suppl):46–56.
39. Sakuma K, Akiho M, Nakashima H, et al. Cyclosporin A modulates cellular localization of MEF2C protein and blocks fiber hypertrophy in the overloaded soleus muscle of mice. Acta Neuropathol 2008;115(6):663–74.
40. Miyabara EH, Aoki MS, Moriscot AS. Cyclosporin A preferentially attenuates skeletal slow-twitch muscle regeneration. Braz J Med Biol Res 2005;38(4): 559–63.
41. Terada S, Nakagawa H, Nakamura Y, et al. Calcineurin is not involved in some mitochondrial enzyme adaptations to endurance exercise training in rat skeletal muscle. Eur J Appl Physiol 2003;90(1-2):210–7.
42. Schmid H, Schmitt H, Eissele R, et al. Nephrotoxicity of cyclosporine A in the rat. Ren Physiol Biochem 1993;16:146–55.
43. Breil M, Chariot P. Muscle disorders associated with cyclosporine treatment. Muscle Nerve 1999;22(12):1631–6.
44. Killian KJ, LeBlanc P, Martin DH, et al. Exercise capacity and ventilatory, circulatory, and symptom limitation in patients with airflow limitation. Am Rev Respir Dis 1992;146:935–40.
45. Mador MJ, Kufel TJ, Piineda L. Quadriceps fatigue following cycle exercise in patients with COPD. Am J Respir Crit Care Med 2000;161:447–53.
46. Bartels MN, Kim H, Whiteson JH, et al. Pulmonary rehabilitation in patients undergoing lung-volume reduction surgery. Arch Phys Med Rehabil 2006;87(3 Suppl): 84–8.
47. Bartels MN. Rehabilitation management of lung volume reduction surgery. In: Ginsburg M, editor. Lung volume reduction surgery. St Louis (MO): Mosby-Year Book, Inc; 2001. p. 97–124.
48. Lederer DJ, Thomashow BM, Ginsburg ME, et al. Lung-volume reduction surgery for pulmonary emphysema: Improvement in body mass index, airflow obstruction, dyspnea, and exercise capacity index after 1 year. J Thorac Cardiovasc Surg 2007;133(6):1434–8.
49. Ries AL, Make BJ, Lee SM, et al. National Emphysema Treatment Trial Research Group. The effects of pulmonary rehabilitation in the national emphysema treatment trial. Chest 2005;128(6):3799–809.
50. King AC, Haskell WL, Taylor CB, et al. Group vs. home-based exercise training in healthy older men and women. JAMA 1991;266:1535–42.
51. Franklin BA, Gordon S, Timmis GC. Amount of exercise necessary for the patient with coronary artery disease. Am J Cardiol 1992;69:1426–32.
52. Pate RR, Pratt M, Blair SN, et al. Physical activity and public health: a recommendation from the Centers for Disease Control and Prevention and the American College of Sports Medicine. JAMA 1995;273:402–7.
53. DeBusk RF, Stenestrand U, Sheehan M, et al. Training effects of long versus short bouts of exercise in healthy subjects. Am J Cardiol 1990;65:1010–3.
54. Franklin BA, Vander L, Wrisley D, et al. Training ability of arms versus legs in men with previous myocardial infarction. Chest 1994;105:262–4.
55. Bartels MN. The role of pulmonary rehabilitation for patients undergoing lung volume reduction surgery. Minerva Pneumologica. Invited Review. Special issue distributed at the Congress of the Italian Society of Respiratory Medicine (Florence, October 4–7). Minerva Pneumol 2006;45:177–96.

56. Alba AS, Kim H, Whiteson JH, et al. Cardiopulmonary rehabilitation and cancer rehabilitation. 2. Pulmonary rehabilitation review. Arch Phys Med Rehabil 2006; 87(3 Suppl):57–64.
57. Franklin BA. Motivating patients to exercise: strategies to increase compliance. Sports Med Digest 1994;16:1–3.
58. American College of Sports Medicine. In: Durstine JL, Bloomquist LE, Figoni SF, et al, editors. ACSM's exercise management for persons with chronic disease and disabilities. 1st edition. Champaign (IL): Human Kinetics; 1997.

Cancer-Related Fatigue

Andrea L. Cheville, MD, MSCE

KEYWORDS

• Cancer • Fatigue • Exercise • Review • Symptom

Cancer-related fatigue (CRF) is a prevalent and morbid etiologic puzzle. Its relevance is demonstrated by the fact that between one-half and one-third of Americans will develop cancer, and >90% of patients will experience CRF at some point in their disease course. Patients describe CRF as devastating to many life domains, degrading their vocational, familial, and societal roles.[1] Patients rate CRF as more distressing than any other cancer- or treatment-related symptom, including pain, with symptoms persisting for years after discontinuation of cancer treatment.[2] CRF is perhaps the single most challenging barrier to effective rehabilitation of cancer patients, because it severely constrains patients' ability to actively engage in functional restoration and adhere to the long-term programs required for success. CRF may become so severe that patients interrupt or abandon cancer treatment.[2]

Despite accord that CRF is an important issue with wide-reaching public health and fiscal consequences, a pithy, simplistic definition that distinguishes CRF from related symptoms and syndromes (eg, chemotherapy-induced anemia, "chemo-brain") remains elusive. Most experts concur that fatigue is a multidimensional experience with physical and cognitive dimensions. Whether and how often physical and/or cognitive features persist when all remediable factors have been definitively addressed (eg, endocrinopathies, depression) is uncertain, hence the ongoing debate regarding the unique features of CRF.

Dishearteningly, despite extensive research, effective primary and secondary preventive strategies remain limited. This lack reflects the investigative challenge of differentiating and measuring fatigue in populations with many relevant and changing characteristics (eg, disease and treatment status, elapsed time since treatment).

DEFINITION

Several definitions have been proposed. All are useful, and the subtle differences between them illustrate extant controversies in the field. The National Consortium of Cancer Centers (NCCN) defines fatigue as, "an unusual persistent subjective sense of tiredness related to cancer or cancer treatment that interferes with usual functioning."[3] Diagnosis of CRF according to the International Classification of Disease (ICD)-10 requires a known tumor and daily persistence of the symptom for ≥ 2 weeks plus 6 of the following 11 complaints: diminished energy, increasing need for rest, limb heaviness,

Department of Physical Medicine and Rehabilitation, Mayo Clinic, 200 First Street SW, Rochester, MN 55944, USA
E-mail address: cheville.andrea@mayo.edu

Phys Med Rehabil Clin N Am 20 (2009) 405–416
doi:10.1016/j.pmr.2008.12.005
1047-9651/08/$ – see front matter

diminished ability to concentrate, decreased interest in engaging in normal activities, sleep disorder, inertia, emotional lability due to fatigue, perceived problems with short-term memory, and postexertional malaise exceeding several hours (**Table 1**).[4]

Although not included in most formal definitions, additional, accepted characteristics of CRF include tiredness disproportionate to the intensity of patients' exertional level, which is not relieved by rest or sleep and subjective weakness.[5–7] Experts concur that fatigue reduces the mental capacity and psychological resilience of cancer patients.[8,9] Psychological complaints may include reduced motivation, capacity to attend, and concentration. Patients may also experience difficulty with new learning.[10]

EPIDEMIOLOGY

Fatigue occurs most commonly and severely during administration of anticancer therapies. CRF is experienced by up to 99% of patients receiving chemotherapy with complaints generally being most intense during the first 3 days after chemotherapy administration and improving gradually over the subsequent week.[11] Over 40% of patients rate their fatigue as "severe" or ≥ 7 on an 11-point numerical rating scale.[12] CRF incidence rates in the clinical trial setting range from 70% to 80%, with variations being explained by differences in cancer and treatment type.[13] CRF is frequently present during diagnosis, increases throughout treatment, and commonly persists for years after the completion of therapy.[10,14] CRF continues to be problematic even when survivors' cancer is undetectable. Reported incidence rates of CRF among cancer survivors range as high as 81%, with 17% to 38% reporting high levels of fatigue during 6 months after treatment.[15,16] Fatigue is associated with decreased disease-free and overall survival among cancer patients.[17]

ASSESSMENT

Symptom characterization is the prime goal of fatigue assessment. However, comprehensive evaluation should address cancer treatment history, medical comorbidities, and associated symptoms. Physical examination may reveal remediable etiologies. An approach to fatigue assessment similar to that endorsed for pain evaluation has been proposed, including use of 11-point numeric rating scales (NRS) to characterize symptom intensity "at worse," "at best," and "on average."[18] NRS can also be used to query patients regarding fatigue interference with work, relations with others, recreational activities, and so on. The responsiveness of fatigue NRS to changes in symptom intensity has been established.

Fatigue is frequently assessed in epidemiologic studies and therapeutic trials using validated multidimensional instruments. Many such instruments are available, and they vary considerably in length. Examples of patient report assessment instruments include the Functional Assessment of Cancer Treatment-Fatigue scale (FACT-F),[19] Profile of Mood States (POMS) vigor and fatigue subscales,[20] Piper Fatigue Scale,[21] and Multidimensional Fatigue Inventory.[22] The length and complex scoring algorithms of many of these instruments limit their utility in clinical practice. However, short forms have been developed for some instruments, for example, POMS Short-Form fatigue subscale. Coadministration with depression and pain assessment tools can help clinicians to unravel the frequent puzzle of concurrent symptoms.

ASSOCIATED SYMPTOMS

Fatigue frequently occurs in association with pain, depression and anxiety, dyspnea, and insomnia, among other symptoms.[23] The strength of the associations varies

Table 1
ICD-10 criteria for cancer-related fatigue
Diminished energy
Increasing need for rest
Limb heaviness
Diminished ability to concentrate
Decreased interest in engaging in normal activities
Sleep disorder
Inertia
Emotional lability due to fatigue
Perceived problems with short-term memory
Postexertional malaise exceeding several hours

depending on the study population, whether patients are receiving active treatment, and patients' cancer stage. The fact that these associations have not been prospectively or longitudinally studied in a broad range of cohorts severely limits any conclusions that can be drawn regarding causal relationships or common etiologies. Clinicians have long appreciated the inciting and sustaining roles that symptoms such as pain can play in the development and persistence of fatigue. Intense, persistent, or refractory symptoms unquestionably engender fatigue. Symptoms may reciprocally intensify each other. For example, depression and fatigue may aggravate each other though arising from different sources. Conversely, in many cases a common pathology, for example, tumors, may produce local symptoms of effects on adjacent bones and nerves while simultaneously elaborating biological response modifiers that produce fatigue.

Most reported associations between CRF and other symptoms are the product of regression modeling of cross-sectional data gleaned from cohorts defined by disease, stage, and treatment status (eg, breast cancer survivors). Few studies have followed cohorts longitudinally. Therefore, little is known about the inter-relationships of symptoms over time. Approximately 19% of patients with CRF are clinically depressed. An estimated 30% to 35% of the variance in fatigue can be attributed to concurrent symptoms, with pain being the most relevant.[24] Dyspnea associates strongly with fatigue in advanced cancer, and along with pain and psychological distress explained 56% of fatigue variance in 1 report.[25] In a different study, pain accounted for 40% of fatigue variance.[26]

The construct of "symptom clusters" has featured prominently in the cancer literature in recent years, with fatigue appearing among many proposed clusters. Investigations are underway to identify genetic factors that may explain cluster patterns; however, such efforts have yet to generate clinically applicable information. Although fatigue clearly associates with adverse symptoms, evidence is inconsistent as to whether symptom control ameliorates CRF. Nonetheless, a comprehensive symptom assessment is warranted in the evaluation of CRF, and effective treatment can be reasonably anticipated to improve fatigue.

REMEDIABLE CONTRIBUTORS

A discrete source and are of of fatigue can be identified in some patients, leading to effective treatment and symptom reversal. Commonly, many potentially contributory mechanisms can be identified and are of uncertain relative importance. Abetting conditions include endocrinopathies (hypogonadism, hypothyroidism, adrenal insuffi-ciency), blood dyscrasia (anemia), degraded sleep quality (obstructive sleep apnea), centrally acting medications, steroid myopathy, and cachexia (**Table 2**). Each of these possibilities should be examined in cancer patients presenting with fatigue; though anemia often receives disproportionate attention.

The historic focus on anemia is understandable, since hemoglobin diminishes in patients receiving antineoplastic therapy. Roughly 50% of patients with solid tumors are anemic at diagnosis.[27] Hematologic malignancies are associated with higher prev-alences; for example, 60% to 70% of patients with non-Hodgkin's lymphoma are anemic at the time of diagnosis.[27] The relevance of anemia to CRF has received less emphasis of late. Initial interest stemmed from reports that fatigue severity paral-leled reductions in serum hemoglobin.[8,28] More recently, it has been appreciated that the time course of fatigue onset and improvement differs substantially from fluctua-tions in blood counts. Normalization of hemoglobin levels through blood transfusion or erythropoietin administration inconsistently alleviates fatigue. Further, physician practices with respect to threshold hemoglobin levels for treatment are inconsistent, ranging from 7.5 g/dL to 10.7 g/dL.[29] This inconsistency reflects the fact that no specific decrement or increment in hemoglobin value has been definitively linked to quantitative changes in quality of life (QOL).

Apart from anemia's role in CRF, no one disputes that even mild anemia can signif-icantly compromise subjective QOL.[30] Hence, proactive treatment with recombinant erythropoietin is widely accepted. The Anemia Guidelines Development Group recom-mends starting epoetins in patients with prechemotherapy baseline hemoglobin of <10 g/dL, symptomatic baseline anemia, or a drop of 1 to 2 g/dL per chemotherapy cycle.[31] The American Society of Clinical Oncology (ASCO)/American Society of Hematology (ASH) guidelines also use 10 g/dL as the threshold hemoglobin value.[32] Patients who have poor responses to epoetin therapy, intensely symptomatic anemia, hemoglobin levels ≤9 g/dL, or economic constraints to epoetin access may require red blood cell transfusion.

Endocrinopathies should be sought due to the frequency of underdiagnosis and the ready availability of replacement therapies. Disruption of the adrenal axis, thyroid gland, testes, and ovaries by chemical ablation, surgical resection, or irradiation can contribute to fatigue. Appropriate serologies will facilitate rapid identification of deficiencies.

| Table 2 |
Comorbidities associated with cancer-related fatigue
Endocrinopathies
Hypogonadism
Hypothyroidism
Adrenal insufficiency
Blood dyscrasia
Anemia
Degraded sleep quality
Obstructive sleep apnea
Centrally acting medications
Steroid myopathy
Cachexia

Other remediable contributors can be expeditiously detected through appropriate assessments. Reports of poor sleep may indicate the need for a sleep study if elimination of daytime napping and use of soporifics are unhelpful. Centrally acting pharmaceuticals should be eliminated or replaced by less problematic alternatives whenever possible. A reduction or withdrawal trial of nonessential drugs can identify those producing fatigue.[9] Although steroid myopathy may be inescapable due to the need for co-administration of steroids with chemotherapy, its timely recognition may permit steroid dose reduction and accurate prognostication, which is appreciated by patients.

Deconditioning related to inactivity is common among cancer patients. If not an instigating factor, deconditioning can aggravate fatigue from other causes. Aerobic exercise, as discussed later, features prominently in the management of CRF. Additionally, exercise contributes to the primary and secondary prevention of breast and colon cancers and perhaps other malignancies as well. Few cancer patients receive formal, practical guidance in how to begin an exercise program. For these reasons, rehabilitation clinicians should provide each patient with concrete, detailed recommendations for an exercise regimen specifying type, intensity, frequency, and plans for program advancement.

PROPOSED MECHANISMS

The pathophysiological processes underlying CRF are incompletely understood. Most proposed mechanisms reflect efforts to account for associations between the intensity of CRF and markers of disease burden, treatment toxicity, symptom burden, and patient behaviors. The elaboration of biological response modifiers (eg, cytokines) by tumors and by the body in response to tumors or treatments was among the earliest explanations. Support derived principally from a well-characterized association between the administration of biological response modifiers for therapeutic purposes and the onset of severe fatigue. Equally suggestive were reports that tumor necrosis factor-α and interleukin-6 are elevated in some patients with chronic fatigue syndrome and that synthetic antibodies directed at proinflammatory cytokines reduce fatigue in patients with rheumatoid arthritis.[33–35] However, efforts to correlate levels of circulating cytokines with CRF have not succeeded.[36] Biological response modifiers, therefore, figure less prominently in current mechanistic discussions, particularly regarding CRF that far outlasts the administration of cancer treatments.

Serotonin (5-HT) dysregulation has been examined as a potential contributor to CRF largely due to mounting evidence that 5-HT plays an important role in disparate fatigue states. 5-HT may contribute to fatigue experienced by healthy subjects during vigorous exercise. Tryptophan is a precursor of 5-HT, and brain tryptophan levels increase significantly during normal exercise.[37] Animal models demonstrate an inverse dose relationship between treadmill endurance and 5-HT.[38] Further, circulating tryptophan levels are elevated in chronic fatigue syndrome.[39] Despite suggestive findings implicating 5-HT, central 5-HT concentrations do not correlate with the presence or intensity of CRF.[40,41]

Data directly link aberrant hypothalamic-pituitary-adrenal (HPA) axis function to CRF, among other sources of fatigue. Breast cancer survivors with CRF have reduced waking serum cortisol levels, relative to their unaffected counterparts.[42] Exposing CRF-afflicted breast cancer survivors to a controlled stressor produced blunted stress responses as reflected in low salivary cortisol levels (**Fig. 1**).[43] The investigators question whether irregularities in diurnal cortisol regulation may ultimately prove more relevant to CRF than overall cortisol levels.[44] The HPA axis has been proposed to be the

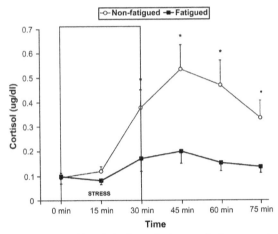

Fig. 1. Mean salivary free cortisol levels before, during, and after experimental psychologic stress in fatigued and nonfatigued breast cancer survivors. The stressor occurred during the first 30 min indicated on the graph. Error bars represent 1 standard error. *P<.05.

means by which cytokines and 5-HT may affect CRF, since cortisol, cytokines, and 5-HT levels cross-regulate one another.[10]

Abnormal sleep-wake cycles and rest-activity patterns were detected in patients with CRF. Using actigraphy to quantify movement, an inverse relationship was demonstrated between daytime physical activity and fatigue in patients with breast and colorectal cancers.[45,46] The converse was true at night, with daytime fatigue correlating directly with excessive movement during sleep. Dampened variation in 24-hour rest-activity patterns associates with fatigue levels among patients with stage IV colorectal cancer.[17,47] Variations in the normality of circadian rhythms of patients receiving adjuvant chemotherapy for breast cancer correlated with changes in fatigue across chemotherapy cycles.[48]

Concerted investigative effort has yet to yield a definitive mechanism, which likely reflects the underlying complexity and nonuniform pathogenesis of CRF. That many of the mechanisms heretofore discussed are interrelated and play dominant roles at different times across the trajectory of cancer diagnosis, treatment, and survivorship is little argued. An important observation for physiatrists is the fact that therapeutic exercise will influence virtually all implicated mechanisms in a salutary fashion. Comprehensive care of all cancer patients should include guidance in formulating an individualized and gently incremental exercise program.

TREATMENT

Given the high level of uncertainty regarding the mechanisms responsible for CRF, treatment approaches are empiric. Once reversible sources of fatigue have been ruled out or treated, a palliative, "symptom-oriented" approach to CRF management is appropriate. A multimodal approach that includes medications, exercise, psychological interventions, and improved sleep hygiene offers the greatest likelihood of success and has been endorsed by the National Comprehensive Cancer Network.[49]

Pharmacologic Approaches

Methylphenidate has been used most extensively to treat fatigue in cancer patients. Seven clinical trials have examined the efficacy of methylphenidate in alleviating CRF. Four open-label studies in mixed cancer cohorts resulted in benefit.[50–53]

A small pilot study combining exercise and methylphenidate was also open label and reported benefit.[54] Results from 2 double-blind studies conflict.[55,56] However, inconsistencies may be due to different maximal doses, trial duration, and inclusion criteria. During a 7-day trial of methylphenidate (maximal dose, 20 mg/d), Bruera and colleagues did not find that methylphenidate reduced CRF to a greater extent than placebo.[55] In contrast, Lower and Cooper[56] excluded anemic patients, titrated methylphenidate to a maximal dose of 50 mg/d, and continued treatment for 2 months. With these study parameters, methylphenidate afforded significant reduction in CRF.[56] Further double-blind studies would be helpful in clarifying treatment parameters and patients most likely to benefit. Until such guidance becomes available, it is reasonable to trial methylphenidate at a starting dose of 5 to 10 mg/d. Dose-limiting toxicities associated with methylphenidate include anorexia, insomnia, anxiety, confusion, tremor, and tachycardia.

Modafinil, also a central nervous system stimulant, has been less rigorously studied in limited open-label trials. In 1 of 2 modafinil trials, breast cancer survivors reported less fatigue even with CRF of up to 2 years' duration.[57] Kaleita and colleagues[58] studied the effects of modafinil in patients with brain tumors, a disparate cohort, and also detected benefit. Modafinil is relatively well tolerated, causing side effects (eg, headache, anxiety, nausea) generally rated as mild, which resolve on discontinuation. Modafinil therapy can be initiated at 100 to 200 mg/d and titrated to a maximal dose of 400 mg/d.

Antidepressants have inconsistently alleviated CRF in depressed cancer patients. Two open-label case series of sustained-release bupropion (100–300 mg/d) detected benefit 2 to 4 weeks after the start of treatment.[59,60] Paroxetine has been more rigorously studied in 2 double-blind trials. The results of both studies revealed improved depression scores but no change in fatigue levels.[40,41] The effect of serotonin-norepinephrine reuptake inhibitors on CRF has yet to be characterized.

The effects of corticosteroids have been rigorously studied in patients with advanced, metastatic cancer and related fatigue. The results of 2 randomized, double-blind, crossover studies demonstrated reduced fatigue; 1 used methylprednisolone and the other megesterol acetate.[61,62] Both studies were of short duration: ≤14 days. Prednisone also reduced fatigue in a less rigorous open-label study.[63] Side effects associated with long-term steroid use may limit its utility to patients with advanced cancer.

Small open-label designs have been used to assess whether L-carnitine reduces CRF. The results of 3 such studies, all with limited sample sizes, have shown benefit.[64–66] Twelve patients with stage III or IV malignancies who were treated for 4 weeks reported diminished fatigue and enhanced QOL.[64] A larger trial, N = 50, restricted enrollment to patients with stage IV cancer.[65] Subjects experienced benefit during 1 week of treatment based on FACT-F scores. Cruciani and colleagues[66] studied 12 patients with mixed tumors and noted a 90% reduction in fatigue. L-carnitine was dosed at 500 to 600 mg/d in all studies. These promising results have yet to be replicated with blinded, controlled study design.

Nonpharmacologic Behavioral Interventions

Exercise, both aerobic and resistive, offers great promise in the alleviation of CRF. Studies in breast cancer patients receiving chemo- or radiation therapy have consistently reported improved symptom burden, particularly fatigue.[67] Encouraging results have been reported in other cancer cohorts. For example, Oldervoll and colleagues[29] exercised patients with Hodgkin's disease post-treatment at 65% to 80% of maximal heart rate for 40 to 60 minutes 3 times/wk and noted marked CRF improvement. Colorectal patients participating in a home-based program of patient-preferred exercise 3 to 5 times/wk at 65% to 75% of maximal heart rate for 20 to 30 minutes also reported decreased fatigue, whereas fatigue increased in members of the control group.[68] No harm has been associated with aerobic exercise at 75% to 80% maximal heart rate.

Resistance training has been more limitedly studied than aerobic exercise, yet the promising pattern of reduced CRF is evident. Segal and colleagues[69] studied androgen-deprived patients with prostate cancer. Upper- and lower-extremity muscle groups were trained with 2 sets of 8 to 12 repetitions at 60% to 70% of heart rate and 1 maximal repetition over a 12-week program. Postexercise assessment revealed improved QOL, fatigue, and strength. Campbell and colleagues[70] used a mixed aerobic and resistive training approach to study patients with breast cancer. CRF diminished to a greater extent among participants in the exercise relative to those in the control group. No study has reported compromised QOL associated with participation in exercise programs, irrespective of their intensity. The impact of exercise on QOL does not correlate with either program intensity or the magnitude of physiologic training effect, suggesting that the clinicians should strongly endorse exercise of any form and intensity.

The overall positive effect of exercise on CRF is now accepted as fact. It is worth noting that recruitment for exercise protocols is challenging, which likely stems from patient-based barriers to exercise. Many patients have limited access to supervised, structured exercise programs or exercise facilities; thus, identifying some feasible means by which patients can engage in regular full-body movement of any type is a laudable starting point. Opportunities to "exercise" that integrate social support, relaxation, positive atmosphere, and other reinforcing factors have been inadequately studied. This deficit is problematic, since long-term adherence to exercise programs, even among patients who derive unequivocal benefit, is limited.

A growing body of evidence also supports the use of psychosocial interventions to mitigate CRF. Randomized, controlled study designs have been used to assess the effect of a wide variety of interventions on CRF. Studied cohorts have varied considerably with respect to cancer type, stage, and treatment status. Interventions have been equally disparate, including support groups, psychoeducational nursing interventions (eg, coping, stress management, problem solving), energy conservation and activity management, psychologist- or self-administered stress management, nurse-administered cognitive behavioral symptom management intervention, structured psychiatric group intervention, audiotape played before treatment, and so on.[14] A consistent pattern of CRF reduction is found across this broad array of therapeutic approaches. Unfortunately, despite strong supportive evidence, such programs are not routinely available outside of research studies. If readers can avail their patients of such services, it is certainly worthwhile to do so with the caveat that intensive and demanding programs can actually worsen CRF.[71]

SUMMARY

CRF is indisputably a significant problem with important public health and medical economic implications. As the prevalence of cancer survivorship grows, the impact of CRF will increase. Physiatrists have not historically played an active role in caring for affected patients. In the author's opinion, this is unfortunate, since the holistic, integrated, and cross-disciplinary approach that characterizes physiatry seems ideally suited to offer patients meaningful benefit. Physiatrists with a clinical interest are likely to be robustly rewarded with interest from the oncological community, as CRF is a frustrating and devastating problem for patients and clinicians alike.

REFERENCES

1. Curt GA, Breitbart W, Cella D, et al. Impact of cancer-related fatigue on the lives of patients: new findings from the fatigue coalition. Oncologist 2000;5(5):353–60.
2. Hofman M, Ryan JL, Figueroa-Moseley CD, et al. Cancer-related fatigue: the scale of the problem. Oncologist 2007;12(Suppl 1):4–10.
3. Mock V, Atkinson A, Barsevick A, et al. NCCN practice guidelines for cancer-related fatigue. Oncology (Williston Park) 2000;14(11A):151–61.
4. World Health Organization. International statistical classification of diseases and related health problems 1989 revision. Geneva: World Health Organization; 2003.
5. Ahlberg K, Ekman T, Gaston-Johansson F, et al. Assessment and management of cancer-related fatigue in adults. Lancet 2003;362(9384):640–50.
6. Morrow GR, Hickok JT, Andrews PL, et al. Reduction in serum cortisol after platinum based chemotherapy for cancer: a role for the HPA axis in treatment-related nausea? Psychophysiology 2002;39(4):491–5.
7. Morrow GR, Andrews PL, Hickok JT, et al. Fatigue associated with cancer and its treatment. Support Care Cancer 2002;10(5):389–98.
8. Cella D. Factors influencing quality of life in cancer patients: anemia and fatigue. Semin Oncol 1998;25(3 Suppl 7):43–6.
9. Miaskowski C. The need to assess multiple symptoms. Pain Manag Nurs 2002; 3(4):115.
10. Ryan JL, Carroll JK, Ryan EP, et al. Mechanisms of cancer-related fatigue. Oncologist 2007;12(Suppl 1):22–34.
11. Schwartz AL, Nail LM, Chen S, et al. Fatigue patterns observed in patients receiving chemotherapy and radiotherapy. Cancer Invest 2000;18(1):11–9.
12. Hickok JT, Roscoe JA, Morrow GR, et al. Frequency, severity, clinical course, and correlates of fatigue in 372 patients during 5 weeks of radiotherapy for cancer. Cancer 2005;104(8):1772–8.
13. Lawrence DP, Kupelnick B, Miller K, et al. Evidence report on the occurrence, assessment, and treatment of fatigue in cancer patients. J Natl Cancer Inst Monographs 2004;32:40–50.
14. Mustian KM, Morrow GR, Carroll JK, et al. Integrative nonpharmacologic behavioral interventions for the management of cancer-related fatigue. Oncologist 2007;12(Suppl 1):52–67.
15. Fobair P, Hoppe RT, Bloom J, et al. Psychosocial problems among survivors of Hodgkin's disease. J Clin Oncol 1986;4(5):805–14.
16. Prue G, Rankin J, Allen J, et al. Cancer-related fatigue: a critical appraisal. Eur J Cancer 2006;42(7):846–63.
17. Mormont MC, Waterhouse J, Bleuzen P, et al. Marked 24-h rest/activity rhythms are associated with better quality of life, better response, and longer survival in patients with metastatic colorectal cancer and good performance status. Clin Cancer Res 2000;6(8):3038–45.
18. Mendoza TR, Wang XS, Cleeland CS, et al. The rapid assessment of fatigue severity in cancer patients: use of the brief fatigue inventory. Cancer 1999; 85(5):1186–96.

19. Yellen SB, Cella DF, Webster K, et al. Measuring fatigue and other anemia-related symptoms with the Functional Assessment of Cancer Therapy (FACT) measurement system. J Pain Symptom Manage 1997;13(2):63–74.
20. McNair Dm LM, Droppleman LF. Profile of mood states [Revised]. San Diego (CA): EdITS/Educational and Industrial Testing Service; 1992.
21. Piper BF, Dibble SL, Dodd MJ, et al. The revised piper fatigue scale: psychometric evaluation in women with breast cancer. Oncol Nurs Forum 1998;25(4):677–84.
22. Smets EM, Garssen B, Bonke B, et al. The Multidimensional Fatigue Inventory (MFI) psychometric qualities of an instrument to assess fatigue. J Psychosom Res 1995;39(3):315–25.
23. Davidson JR, MacLean AW, Brundage MD, et al. Sleep disturbance in cancer patients. Soc Sci Med 2002;54(9):1309–21.
24. Bower JE. Prevalence and causes of fatigue after cancer treatment: the next generation of research. J Clin Oncol 2005;23(33):8280–2.
25. Stone P, Richards M, A'Hern R, et al. A study to investigate the prevalence, severity and correlates of fatigue among patients with cancer in comparison with a control group of volunteers without cancer. Ann Oncol 2000;11(5):561–7.
26. Given B, Given CW, McCorkle R, et al. Pain and fatigue management: results of a nursing randomized clinical trial. Oncol Nurs Forum 2002;29(6):949–56.
27. Bohlius J, Weingart O, Trelle S, et al. Cancer-related anemia and recombinant human erythropoietin–an updated overview. Nat Clin Pract Oncol 2006;3(3): 152–64.
28. Curt GA. Impact of fatigue on quality of life in oncology patients. Semin Hematol 2000;37(4 Suppl 6):14–7.
29. Oldervoll LM, Kaasa S, Knobel H, et al. Exercise reduces fatigue in chronic fatigued Hodgkin's disease survivors–results from a pilot study. Eur J Cancer 2003;39(1):57–63.
30. Lucca U, Tettamanti M, Mosconi P, et al. Association of mild anemia with cognitive, functional, mood and quality of life outcomes in the elderly: the "Health and Anemia" study. PLoS ONE 2008;3(4):e1920.
31. Turner R, Anglin P, Burkes R, et al. Epoetin alfa in cancer patients: evidence-based guidelines. J Pain Symptom Manage 2001;22(5):954–65.
32. Rizzo JD, Somerfield MR, Hagerty KL, et al. Use of epoetin and darbepoetin in patients with cancer: 2007 American Society of Clinical Oncology/American Society of Hematology clinical practice guideline update. J Clin Oncol 2008; 26(1):132–49.
33. Chao CC, Gallagher M, Phair J, et al. Serum neopterin and interleukin-6 levels in chronic fatigue syndrome. J Infect Dis 1990;162(6):1412–3.
34. Patarca R, Klimas NG, Lugtendorf S, et al. Dysregulated expression of tumor necrosis factor in chronic fatigue syndrome: interrelations with cellular sources and patterns of soluble immune mediator expression. Clin Infect Dis 1994; 18(Suppl 1):S147–53.
35. Weinblatt ME, Keystone EC, Furst DE, et al. Adalimumab, a fully human anti-tumor necrosis factor alpha monoclonal antibody, for the treatment of rheumatoid arthritis in patients taking concomitant methotrexate: the ARMADA trial. Arthritis Rheum 2003;48(1):35–45.
36. Pusztai L, Mendoza TR, Reuben JM, et al. Changes in plasma levels of inflammatory cytokines in response to paclitaxel chemotherapy. Cytokines 2004;25(3): 94–102.
37. Fernstrom JD, Fernstrom MH. Exercise, serum free tryptophan, and central fatigue. J Nutr 2006;136(2):553S–9S.

38. Bailey SP, Davis JM, Ahlborn EN. Effect of increased brain serotonergic activity on endurance performance in the rat. Acta Physiol Scand 1992;145(1):75–6.
39. Badawy AA, Morgan CJ, Llewelyn MB, et al. Heterogeneity of serum tryptophan concentration and availability to the brain in patients with the chronic fatigue syndrome. J Psychopharmacol 2005;19(4):385–91.
40. Morrow GR, Hickok JT, Roscoe JA, et al. Differential effects of paroxetine on fatigue and depression: a randomized, double-blind trial from the University of Rochester cancer center community clinical oncology program. J Clin Oncol 2003;21(24):4635–41.
41. Roscoe JA, Morrow GR, Hickok JT, et al. Effect of paroxetine hydrochloride (Paxil) on fatigue and depression in breast cancer patients receiving chemotherapy. Breast Cancer Res Treat 2005;89(3):243–9.
42. Bower JE, Ganz PA, Aziz N, et al. Fatigue and proinflammatory cytokine activity in breast cancer survivors. Psychosom Med 2002;64(4):604–11.
43. Bower JE, Ganz PA, Aziz N. Altered cortisol response to psychologic stress in breast cancer survivors with persistent fatigue. Psychosom Med 2005;67(2):277–80.
44. Bower JE, Ganz PA, Dickerson SS, et al. Diurnal cortisol rhythm and fatigue in breast cancer survivors. Psychoneuroendocrinology 2005;30(1):92–100.
45. Mormont MC, De Prins J, Levi F. [Study of circadian rhythms of activity by actometry: preliminary results in 30 patients with metastatic colorectal cancer] [French]. Pathol Biol (Paris) 1996;44(3):165–71.
46. Mormont MC, Hecquet B, Bogdan A, et al. Non-invasive estimation of the circadian rhythm in serum cortisol in patients with ovarian or colorectal cancer. Int J Cancer 1998;78(4):421–4.
47. Rich T, Innominato PF, Boerner J, et al. Elevated serum cytokines correlated with altered behavior, serum cortisol rhythm, and dampened 24-hour rest-activity patterns in patients with metastatic colorectal cancer. Clin Cancer Res 2005;11(5):1757–64.
48. Roscoe JA, Morrow GR, Hickok JT, et al. Temporal interrelationships among fatigue, circadian rhythm and depression in breast cancer patients undergoing chemotherapy treatment. Support Care Cancer 2002;10(4):329–36.
49. (NCCN) Nccn. Clinical practice guidelines in oncology: cancer-related fatigue, v1. Available at: http://www.nccn.org/professionals/physician_glf/PDF/fatigue.pdf. Accessed November 30, 2008.
50. Bruera E, Driver L, Barnes EA, et al. Patient-controlled methylphenidate for the management of fatigue in patients with advanced cancer: a preliminary report. J Clin Oncol 2003;21(23):4439–43.
51. Sarhill N, Walsh D, Nelson KA, et al. Methylphenidate for fatigue in advanced cancer: a prospective open-label pilot study. Am J Hosp Palliat Care 2001;18(3):187–92.
52. Homsi J, Nelson KA, Sarhill N, et al. A phase II study of methylphenidate for depression in advanced cancer. Am J Hosp Palliat Care 2001;18(6):403–7.
53. Hanna A, Sledge G, Mayer ML, et al. A phase II study of methylphenidate for the treatment of fatigue. Support Care Cancer 2006;14(3):210–5.
54. Schwartz AL, Thompson JA, Masood N. Interferon-induced fatigue in patients with melanoma: a pilot study of exercise and methylphenidate. Oncol Nurs Forum 2002;29(7):E85–90.
55. Bruera E, Valero V, Driver L, et al. Patient-controlled methylphenidate for cancer fatigue: a double-blind, randomized, placebo-controlled trial. J Clin Oncol 2006;24(13):2073–8.

56. Lower E, Fleishman S, Cooper A, et al. A phase III, randomized placebo-controlled trial of the safety and efficacy of d-MPH as a new treatment of fatigue and "chemobrain" in adult cancer patients. J Clin Oncol 2005 [ASCO] Meeting Abstract 8000.

57. Morrow GR, Gillies LJ OW, Hickok JT, et al. The positive effect of the psycho-stimulant modafinil on fatigue from cancer that persists after treatment is completed. J Clin Oncol 2005 [ASCO Meeting Abstract 8012].

58. Kaleita TA, Wellisch DK, Graham CA, et al. Pilot study of modafinil for treatment of neurobehavioral dysfunction and fatigue in adult patients with brain tumors. J Clin Oncol 2006 [ASCO Meeting Abstract 1503].

59. Cullum JL, Wojciechowski AE, Pelletier G, et al. Bupropion sustained release treatment reduces fatigue in cancer patients. Can J Psychiatry 2004;49(2):139–44.

60. Moss EL, Simpson JS, Pelletier G, et al. An open-label study of the effects of bupropion SR on fatigue, depression and quality of life of mixed-site cancer patients and their partners. Psychooncology 2006;15(3):259–67.

61. Bruera E, Roca E, Cedaro L, et al. Action of oral methylprednisolone in terminal cancer patients: a prospective randomized double-blind study. Cancer Treat Rep 1985;69(7–8):751–4.

62. Bruera E, Ernst S, Hagen N, et al. Effectiveness of megestrol acetate in patients with advanced cancer: a randomized, double-blind, crossover study. Cancer Prev Control 1998;2(2):74–8.

63. Tannock I, Gospodarowicz M, Meakin W, et al. Treatment of metastatic prostatic cancer with low-dose prednisone: evaluation of pain and quality of life as pragmatic indices of response. J Clin Oncol 1989;7(5):590–7.

64. Gramignano G, Lusso MR, Madeddu C, et al. Efficacy of l-carnitine administration on fatigue, nutritional status, oxidative stress, and related quality of life in 12 advanced cancer patients undergoing anticancer therapy. Nutrition 2006;22(2):136–45.

65. Graziano F, Bisonni R, Catalano V, et al. Potential role of levocarnitine supplementation for the treatment of chemotherapy-induced fatigue in non-anaemic cancer patients. Br J Cancer 2002;86(12):1854–7.

66. Cruciani RA, Dvorkin E, Homel P, et al. L-carnitine supplementation for the treatment of fatigue and depressed mood in cancer patients with carnitine deficiency: a preliminary analysis. Ann N Y Acad Sci 2004;1033:168–76.

67. McNeely ML, Campbell KL, Rowe BH, et al. Effects of exercise on breast cancer patients and survivors: a systematic review and meta-analysis. CMAJ 2006;175(1):34–41.

68. Courneya KS, Friedenreich CM, Quinney HA, et al. A randomized trial of exercise and quality of life in colorectal cancer survivors. Eur J Cancer Care (Engl) 2003;12(4):347–57.

69. Segal RJ, Reid RD, Courneya KS, et al. Resistance exercise in men receiving androgen deprivation therapy for prostate cancer. J Clin Oncol 2003;21(9):1653–9.

70. Campbell A, Mutrie N, White F, et al. A pilot study of a supervised group exercise programme as a rehabilitation treatment for women with breast cancer receiving adjuvant treatment. Eur J Oncol Nurs 2005;9(1):56–63.

71. Brown P, Clark MM, Atherton P, et al. Will improvement in quality of life (QOL) impact fatigue in patients receiving radiation therapy for advanced cancer? Am J Clin Oncol 2006;29(1):52–8.

Index

Note: Page numbers of article titles are in **boldface** type.

A

Alcohol Use Disorders Identification Test, 318
Amantadine, for fatigue, 356
   MS-related, 368
Amitriptyline, for fatigue, 356
   fibromyalgia-related, 378
Antidepressants
   for CRF, 411
   tricyclic, for fatigue, 356
Anxiety, fatigue in cardiopulmonary disease and, 394
Arthritis, rheumatoid, fatigue in, 380–381
   exercise for, 382–383
Aspirin, for MS-related fatigue, 368
Atomoxetine, tricyclic, 356

B

Barroso Fatigue Scale, 316–317
Beck Depression Inventory-II, 318
Behavioral therapy, in fatigue management, 357–358
Bracing, for rheumatoid arthritis, 382–383
Bupropion, for CRF, 411

C

CAGE questionnaire, 318
Cancer Fatigue Scale, 319
Cancer-related fatigue (CRF), 319, **405–416**
   assessment of, 406
   comorbidities associated with, 408
   defined, 405–406
   described, 405
   epidemiology of, 406
   proposed mechanisms of, 409–410
   remediable contributors to, 407–409
   symptoms associated with, 406–407
   treatment of, 410–412
   nonpharmacologic behavioral interventions, 411–412
   pharmacologic, 411
Cardiac disease, fatigue in, assessment of, 390–392

Phys Med Rehabil Clin N Am 20 (2009) 417–423
doi:10.1016/S1047-9651(09)00010-2
1047-9651/09/$ – see front matter © 2009 Elsevier Inc. All rights reserved.

pmr.theclinics.com

Moving?

Make sure your subscription moves with you!

To notify us of your new address, find your **Clinics Account Number** (located on your mailing label above your name), and contact customer service at:

E-mail: elspcs@elsevier.com

800-654-2452 (subscribers in the U.S. & Canada)
314-453-7041 (subscribers outside of the U.S. & Canada)

Fax number: 314-523-5170

Elsevier Periodicals Customer Service
11830 Westline Industrial Drive
St. Louis, MO 63146

*To ensure uninterrupted delivery of your subscription, please notify us at least 4 weeks in advance of move.

ELSEVIER

Printed and bound by CPI Group (UK) Ltd, Croydon, CR0 4YY

03/10/2024

01040465-0010